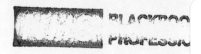

Cross-cultural Psychiatry:
A Practical Guide

Cross-cultural Psychiatry: A Practical Guide

Dinesh Bhugra MA MSc MB BS MPhil FRCPsych PhD

Senior Lecturer in Psychiatry, Institute of Psychiatry, London, UK

Kamaldeep Bhui BSc MSc MB BS MRCPsych MD Dip Clin Psychotherapy

Senior Lecturer in Social & Epidemiological Psychiatry, St Bartholomew's and Royal London Medical and Dental School, London, UK

A member of the Hodder Headline Group
LONDON
Co-published in the USA by Oxford University Press Inc., New York

First published in Great Britain in 2001 by
Arnold, a member of the Hodder Headline Group,
338 Euston Road, London NW1 3BH

http://www.arnoldpublishers.com

Co-published in the USA by
Oxford University Press Inc.,
198 Madison Avenue, New York, NY10016
Oxford is a registered trademark of Oxford University Press

Whilst the advice and information in this book are believed to be true and
accurate at the date of going to press, neither the authors nor the publisher
can accept any legal responsibility or liability for any errors or omissions
that may be made. In particular (but without limiting the generality of the
preceding disclaimer) every effort has been made to check drug dosages;
however, it is still possible that errors have been missed. Furthermore,
dosage schedules are constantly being revised and new side-effects
recognized. For these reasons the reader is strongly urged to consult the
drug companies' printed instructions before administering any of the drugs
recommended in this book.

British Library Cataloguing in Publication Data
A catalogue record for this book is available from the British Library

Library of Congress Cataloging-in-Publication Data
A catalog record for this book is available from the Library of Congress

ISBN 0 340 76379 5

1 2 3 4 5 6 7 8 9 10

Publisher: Georgina Bentliff
Production Editor: Anke Ueberberg
Production Controller: Bryan Eccleshall

Composition by Saxon Graphics Ltd, Derby
Printed and bound in Great Britain by Redwood Books Ltd, Trowbridge

What do you think about this book? Or any other Arnold title?
Please send your comments to feedback.arnold@hodder.co.uk

Contents

Foreword

This new guide is an important route finder for psychiatrists and mental health service professionals who need to find their way through the complexities of mental health service provision in a multicultural society. Specifically, it will be a useful resource for those planning courses in cultural competence and cultural sensitivity, and it will allow educators to develop and then evaluate this crucial educational process. The Royal College of Psychiatrists insists that training in transcultural psychiatry and cultural competence, for example, becomes a core requirement for trainees, as well as for consultants in continuing professional development.

Both authors have proven academic knowledge and experience of cross-cultural dimensions of psychiatry, and this enables them to give readers valuable guidance in this field. Not so long ago there were only few such texts, and the subject was marginalised. Now there is an increasing body of resource materials for educators, and the subject is central to government strategy for the service provision in the National Health Service.

I hope this text will facilitate the black and ethnic minority users to 'come in from the cold' and work with us to develop mental health services for the benefit of all. Within this field we always learn, if we listen, from those who seek our help. Transcultural psychiatry remains a component of routine psychiatric practice and, as H. B. Murphy wrote, it 'begins at home'.

I found this practical text a useful guide to understanding the terrain that all clinicians have to negotiate. It will provoke much-needed research in this field from both the basic sciences and health services research traditions, and it will encourage educators to assess their course and demonstrate that new knowledge, skills and attitudes have been acquired.

John Cox
President
Royal College of Psychiatrists

Introduction

Cross-cultural or comparative psychiatry is the study of the relations between psychiatric disorder and the psychological traits and characteristics of people, the cultures and societies they come from and the interaction between various factors arising from this. Although comparative psychiatry was originally put forward as an academic discipline, it is essential that any academic findings and views are put into practice in the delivery of health care to people from ethnic minorities and even to people belonging to ethnic majority groups different from those to which the clinicians themselves belong. Such an approach takes into account factors which may well be ignored by the researchers and clinicians who work only within single cultures and societies.

Britain is a multicultural society although ethnic minority individuals still make up less than 10 per cent of the population. However, compared with other countries, the needs of ethnic minority groups have been ignored by researchers, clinicians and service providers alike. The impact of processes of migration, subsequent racism (individual and institutional), socio-economic disadvantage and discrimination, social, educational and economic expectations and achievements have been known to play a role in the genesis of one or more mental health disorders, although the research evidence is patchy and mixed. What is apparent, however, is the poor response of some kinds of mental illness to certain treatments. The varying responses to different treatments can be attributed to inappropriate diagnosis, inappropriate management and social and cultural factors. Patients do not always fit into neat categories, either in terms of their mental illness or their ethnicity or culture. Hence clinicians, whatever their discipline, have to be aware of differences as well as similarities between cultures.

We argue that cultural psychiatry is that branch of psychiatry which deals with cultural factors in the genesis and management of psychiatric disorders. The incidence of various psychiatric disorders differs across cultural and ethnic groups. The reasons for varying incidence and prevalence rates can be explained through biological, psychological and social factors. Increasingly the emphasis is beginning to shift from exotic culture-bound syndromes to more culture dependent syndromes. In addition, migration, cultural identity, concepts of the self and childhood and adult attachment, social networks and population density are some of the key factors which may help explain some of the differences in prevalence rates.

For a health professional it is vital that any diagnosis is made in a culturally sensitive and appropriate way. The role of culture in highlighting as well as leading the psychopathology in an individual needs to be understood in the context of social and personal stigma. Family, gender, social expectations and achievement all play a role in help-seeking and compliance. The pathways into care and help-seeking depend upon a number of factors including culture, access to services, provision of services and their availability and explanatory models as they are conceived by the patients and their carers. Idioms of distress will vary according to education, social class, cultural factors and past knowledge and experiences. Thus it becomes crucial for the mental health professional to be aware of some of the pitfalls.

In this volume we have put together a series of assessment and management strategies. We have deliberately not targeted one specific cultural group – we believe that general principles are far more important for understanding issues of cultural assessment. These are as relevant for mental health professionals who belong to the majority culture and deal with patients and carers from minority cultures as they are to mental health professionals who are from minority cultures and are involved in providing care to individuals from majority cultures.

The principles of cultural psychiatry rely on a number of disciplines since psychiatry is perhaps the most multi-disciplinary of all branches of medicine. In addition, social sciences, such as anthropology and its disciplines, such as medical anthropology, social anthropology or critical anthropology and sociology with branches such as medical sociology, have contributed a tremendous amount to the discussion and debate within psychiatry. We have taken some of these ideas on board. We do not aim for this volume to be comprehensive or to be applied blindly to all ethnic groups. We urge the reader to develop their own strategies in innovative ways, using some or all of the strategies set down in this volume. We do not feel that we have all the answers or even most of the answers but hopefully we have opened the doors for clinicians and other health professionals to start thinking seriously about differences and similarities across cultures and individuals.

We thank Melanie Tait at Butterworth-Heinemann and Anke Ueberberg at Arnold for their support, help and encouragement in seeing this project through.

Dinesh Bhugra
Kamaldeep Bhui

Clinical assessment of patients

Introduction

The rates of different types of mental illness vary across different ethnic groups. For example, there is considerable research evidence to suggest that the incidence of schizophrenia in African-Caribbeans in the UK is higher than in the Caribbean (Bhugra *et al.*, 1996, 1997a). Similarly, although some earlier studies suggested that rates of common mental disorders are lower in people from the Indian subcontinent (Brewin, 1980), recent studies have shown that rates are at a par with the indigenous white population but their help-seeking is not at the same level (Jacob *et al.*, 1998). This may suggest that these individuals see their distress as non-medical, and therefore do not seek medical help. This is illustrated in a study where Punjabi women saw depression as part of life's ups and downs, without giving it a medical motif or symbolism (Bhugra *et al.*, 1997b). It is also possible that these individuals may not be aware of the existing services, and that they may seek alternative patterns of care. They may also find that the services do not meet their needs because the providers are unaware of their expressions of distress and the services provided are not culturally sensitive or acceptable. It is possible that in any therapeutic encounter, underlying ignorance of services may play a significant role. In addition, as in most communities, the notion of stigma is high in the minority community's collective mind.

Theoretical background

Psychiatry reflects a system that is dictated by the broader prevalent social, political and economic structures. The availability of and access to health services remains dependent upon political and economic systems. Even when the members of minority ethnic groups seek help, they may well have to cope with individual and institutional racism. The power imbalance within the therapeutic encounter is incredibly important. Therapists, by virtue of their position, experience and training, hold more power, and the therapeutic encounter (although initiated by the patient) is dictated by the professional. The interaction and its implications are shown in Figure 1.1.

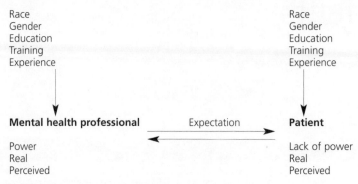

Figure 1.1   The therapeutic encounter.

The basic diagnostic process in psychiatry relies upon observation and assessment of people's behaviour as well as self-reports of emotional state and cognitive processes. The role of cultural factors in the presentation of symptoms and complying with medication must be understood. We do not propose to discuss every cultural factor or every culture, but aim to provide general principles that can be employed across different cultures. By virtue of training, clinicians (whether psychiatrists or nurses) will use a different model from that being employed by patients or their carers. The processes of diagnosis and management do not only include descriptions of symptoms and attempts to identify and deal with the illness; the methods of accessing individual pathology may also be limited. For example, Eisenberg (1977) and Kleinman (1980) have argued that disease as an entity is literally dis-ease, reflecting the underlying psychopathology or pathophysiology, whereas illness is the behaviour which affects others around the patient and is more likely to be dictated by social and cultural factors.

In addition, the nosological systems employed by psychiatry are largely Eurocentric (here we include American models as well, which are Anglocentric) and force clinicians to assume that the mental illnesses commonly found in European patients are to be found in exactly the same way in the non-European patients. Such a universal approach relies on similarities (and indeed looks for these), whereas the presentation of symptoms may well need a relativist approach. A universalist approach is a major problem in that psychiatric disorders that cannot be identified as conforming to the Western diagnostic systems simply appear not to exist. Using acute appendicitis as an example, it is likely that the majority of the patients will complain of pain in the abdomen, some may have vomiting or fever, and on physical examination a tenderness will be noted on

McBurney's point in the vast majority of cases. In a proportion of cases the white blood cell count will be elevated, suggesting an underlying infection. The surgeon may then proceed to appendectomy and the diagnosis confirmed by the pathologist studying the removed appendix. If, on the other hand, a patient presents with vague symptoms of feeling unwell, with palpitations, sweating, diarrhoea etc., this may lead the clinician to look for thyrotoxicosis or malabsorption and a diagnosis of anxiety may be reached by exclusion. Patients may use other terms to express this distress. For example, they may present with 'developing gas' (a term which is very common in North India) or *vai-baadi* (a term used by Punjabis) rather than saying that they feel anxious. A similar example from Taiwan, reported by Kleinman (1980), highlights the problems of differing concepts used by patients and carers on one hand and the health professional on the other. The Chinese patients presented with neurasthenia, and a large proportion of the patients met the criteria for DSM III diagnosis of major depression and as a result were treated with antidepressants. They did get better regarding their mood, but their social functioning did not improve, suggesting that other factors are important in social functioning.

An additional factor that is crucial in successful therapeutic encounters is a mutual position of understanding. The ethnic-minority patient may not perceive the practice of psychiatry as benign. The practice of psychiatry is one way of legitimizing the suppression of non-normative behaviours that may threaten the society. In other words, mental health professionals may well represent the controlling nature of society, which may be perceived as oppressive. An ability to detain patients against their will and then treat them against their will gives a clear message to the community at large, and to members of ethnic communities in particular (Figure 1.2)

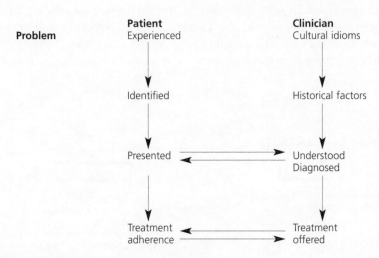

Figure 1.2 Patient–therapist dyad and problems.

In order to understand the relationship between culture and psychopathology, it is essential to recognize psychopathology. The definitions of normal and abnormal are dictated by society, and the agreement within the community regarding what is normal and what is abnormal allows the experts to agree either on phenomenological or statistical norms. In addition, assessment of functioning and social judgement both play a key role in defining abnormality.

The relationship between culture and psychopathology is shown in Figure 1.3. Culture can have a pathoplastic effect on psychopathology; thus, delusions and the contents of hallucinations can be modified according to cultural and prevalent social norms. For example, mustard gas formed a key component of delusions immediately after the Second World War, but it is lasers, Star Trek and similar sci-fi features that play an important part in the current constitution of delusions and hallucinations. Culture-specific syndromes allow the clinician to formulate psychopathology and develop treatment regimens. Culture, when taken to its extreme, can influence overall psychopathology as well as individual symptoms. Prevalence of various conditions can also be influenced by factors other than biological ones.

Psychiatric assessment is not a static or one-sided process, and must take into account social and cultural aspects of distress. The interaction between the patient and the clinician is multilevel, and is illustrated in Figure 1.2. The diagnostic process is two-sided, dynamic and complex, and is influenced by a number of factors.

Language reflects the concerns of a cultural grouping, and certain words may well be specific to some cultures and within that context their meaning is very clear although this may not always be the case. As different cultures place different emphasis on different things related to their survival, clinicians must be sensitive to culture-specific expressions if they are to make sense of idioms of distress. For example, in Hindi there are specific terms for various relationships within the kinship system, whereas in English the terms uncle, aunt or grandparents could reflect a number of relationships. Similarly, various idioms of distress have specific meanings in different

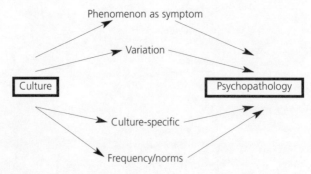

Figure 1.3 Inter-relationship between culture and psychopathology.

cultures. For example, Punjabi women may use the term 'sinking heart' or 'suffering from gas' to describe their symptoms. Tseng (1997) describes the concept of the netting effect in recognizing psychiatric symptoms from the range of psychological expressions, drawing an analogy with fishing nets where different types of net are used to catch different types of fish. This is not to suggest that clinicians should not go on fishing expeditions, but that clinicians must have some previous and existing knowledge of the culture in order to succeed in determining psychopathology.

As long as clinicians are sensitive to differences between cultures and are aware of the possible effects of culture on psychopathology and development of services, they will be more likely to search for and understand human behaviour from the cultural aspect as well as from other perspectives.

Migration

Not all members of minority ethnic groups are likely to be migrants, but some key factors in history and assessment must be remembered. A migrant is an individual who changes a place of residence for any purpose or for any period of time. Technically, visitors for any length of time or students may count as migrants. Groups of migrants may move singly or *en masse*, depending upon their reasons; the politically expelled or refugees may move in groups, whereas economic migrants may move singly and then get their families to join them at a later date. In addition, cultural differences between their original place of residence and the new place may be minimal or extreme, and may include religious, linguistic and social differences. Migrants may not all be rich, successful and enterprising, and may not entirely reflect the population they originate from.

Migration has occurred throughout the history of humankind, and the reasons for it have been economic, social, political, or for personal development. Significant migration in the UK started in the nineteenth century, and after the Second World War the post-war refugee influx occurred. In the 1960s migrant workers were actively recruited to fill low-paid posts and, because of the common language, the recruitment process was relatively easy. At the same time, recruitment from the Indian subcontinent meant that large numbers of males moved to the UK. Their initial hopes were based on economic improvement, suggesting that once they were economically prosperous they would go back. Around the same period, Idi Amin expelled a significant number of Ugandan Asians who migrated *en masse* to the UK. This mass migration led to changes in the immigration law, and it therefore became urgent that families should be brought over before the new laws came into force. Hence the nature of the migration process changed dramatically.

Migrants can be classified according to their reason for migration, the duration of migration or the mobility of migration, whether it is national, international or urban–rural. The distance and attributes of migration are also taken into account in classification. The duration of relocation, voluntary nature of migration and socio-demographic features (such as students or diplomats) may be important in understanding the impact of migration on an individual's psychological functioning. All these factors are also important in understanding the processes of acculturation, which are further described below. Geographical distance from the place of origin influences the frequency of visits and contact with family, and will determine the level and quality of social support. Those who migrate with the intention of settling down will have different sets of problems and expectations to those people who have been forced to migrate, and the former may well have a clearer indication of what to expect and a greater desire to assimilate than the latter. Duration of relocation remains an important variable in ascertaining the period of readjustment, as well as the likelihood of social maladaptations and psychiatric disorders.

Acculturation

Acculturation is a cultural change, initiated by two or more cultural systems, whereby an individual selectively adopts cultural values from another culture (which tends to be dominant). The other extreme of this process is a sense of alienation, which is defined as a sense of not belonging and not feeling welcome. Alienation consists of several features, including a sense of powerlessness, purposelessness, conflict, a sense of social isolation, meaninglessness and self-entrapment. The psychosocial changes experienced and reported by immigrants include assimilation, acculturation, deculturation and absorption.

Assimilation is the process of adjustment, which occurs as a result of two different cultures coming into contact with each other over a prolonged period. Here the individual may acquire the attitudes of other groups and, through sharing of their history and experience, may well be absorbed into a common cultural theme. Assimilation is generally seen as a one-way process.

Acculturation is the process by which an individual undergoes change by contact with the dominant culture, and also as a result of general acculturative change in the broader cultural group. Thus, although acculturation works on the individual, the process may occur at both individual and group levels. In understanding the process of acculturation, various components have to be taken into account. These include identification, and cultural, structural, marital, civic and receptional (encountering prejudice or not prejudice) behaviour. Acculturation can be measured in four dimensions; integration, separation, assimilation and marginalization. When assessing an individual different areas of psychological functioning have to be conceptualized, and these include language, cognitive style, personality traits, individual identity, attitudes and acculturative stress. These characteristics are relatively easy to measure, but a note of caution is indicated: it is important that change (acculturative or otherwise) is measured across the cultural group as well. This is for two reasons. First, it will allow a sense of belonging to the group on behalf of the individual who may well feel alienated from his/her own cultural group, thereby making a lack of social support more likely. Secondly, such a measurement will allow a level of understanding of institutional change and structural variations, as well as socio-political change across structures. Often such an assessment is difficult to measure in clinical practice, but it is essential to do so. It is not only the non-dominant culture that will change; it is possible that such an interaction will influence the dominant culture as well. Culture and personality traits interact very closely, and therefore it is easy to confuse the two. It is also likely that individuals, if feeling threatened by the majority or dominant culture, will become more isolationist or withdraw into their own group. Four acculturative styles – assimilation, integration, marginalizational and ethnocentric coping – may be seen, and each of these has implications for developing understanding of models of illness and pathways into care.

Generational differences

As mentioned earlier, not all migrants will be from minority ethnic groups, and not all ethnic minority individuals will be migrants. It is essential that clinicians are aware of the heterogeneity and differences within groups. The children (even when adults) of migrants will have retained some aspects of their own culture and are also likely to have absorbed some aspects of the majority culture. These assimilations may produce some degree of culture conflict, but this is by no means universal. For example, not all young Asians are likely to be traditional in their views, or to be involved in culture conflict either. A key feature to bear in mind is the fluidity of the culture – no culture remains static, and as culture influences people, people continue to influence culture. There have been suggestions that some mental illnesses are more common in younger generations; hence the clinician must steer away from stereotypical rationalizations and judgements. Some of these differences may be attributed to genetic influences and others to social factors, including cultural identity, acculturation, acculturative stress, prejudice and racism (see Chapter 4).

Thus a composite picture of broader cultural and social factors on one hand, and their interaction with individuals on the other, starts to emerge, and mental health professionals must do everything possible in their grasp to understand cultural mores, taboos, rites of passage and rituals.

Practical implications

Cultural factors act as determinants of need and help seeking. Other social factors such as age, socio-economic status and educational background may well overshadow the racial identity of the individual, especially as communication barriers. Under these circumstances, if cultural variables are over-emphasized the interviewer may be seen as guilty of stereotyping the patient, while if racial and cultural considerations are under-emphasized the clinician may be regarded as guilty of insensitivity to influences that influence the dynamics of the interview (Pederson and Lefley, 1986).

Under these circumstances, clinical competency of clinicians lies in three areas:

1. The beliefs and attitudinal competency of the doctor, including an awareness of his or her own cultural beliefs, heritage, biases and values.

2. A sound understanding and knowledge of the social structure of minority ethnic groups and the institutional barriers they may be facing in coming to seek help.

3. Awareness of verbal and non-verbal communication, and the ability to understand the primacy of one over the other.

These competencies are based on a common-sense approach in the doctor/patient or therapist/client interaction.

Psychiatric assessment

Like all psychiatric assessments, the first interview is just that – the first step – and is the starting point in understanding patients' and their carers' emotional distress and developing a collaborative therapeutic relationship. The aim is not to rush into a diagnosis, which should not be seen as the final stage of the consultation process but as a first step in building a collaborative therapeutic relationship.

If the patient's and clinician's first languages differ, uncertainty about idioms of distress may well inject a sense of confusion and misunderstanding. In addition, quick applications of medical models may lead to inappropriate conclusions. Irrespective of ethnicity, there will be some patients who will require a prolonged period of assessment before a comprehensive management plan can be formulated for optimal intervention. Box 1.1 illustrates the steps required in setting up a clinical assessment.

Communication and cultural distance

As mentioned above, both verbal and non-verbal communication are essential in making sense of a patient's experiences. A sensitive and safe

Box 1.1 Setting up clinical assessment

- Be aware of your limits, competencies, strengths and weaknesses
- Be aware of how your culture has influenced your skills and strengths
- Be aware of patients' and their carers' limitations
- Know the strengths of patients' cultures
- Know the strengths of your culture and how this interacts with patients' cultures
- Know and explore the families' and carers' strengths and weaknesses, especially if they appear to be idiosyncratic
- Assure confidentiality
- Check and double-check the terms used by patients and their carers – make sure you understand them
- Identify idioms of distress
- Assume nothing about the patient

approach is indicated. Prior to setting up the assessment, it is essential that the clinician is aware of basic rudiments of culture such as cultural taboos, rites of passage etc. If the patient's preferred language is not English, the clinician must make arrangements to have a suitable and experienced interpreter present to carry out the interpretation. Only under exceptional circumstances (such as where getting a professional interpreter will cause an inordinate delay in assessment) should family members be used. A professional experienced interpreter can work as a culture broker, teaching and informing the therapist and the therapeutic team and the community as well. Even when the therapist and the clinician speak the same language, it does not necessarily lead to understanding. It has been suggested that clear differences in conversational styles may be seen between different ethnic groups speaking the same language. The clinicians may well benefit from an unstructured period of emotional orientation with the patients and their carers so that key words expressing emotional distress can be identified.

Essential historical data

ADVERSE EVENTS

The clinician must be aware that all life events will have varying significance for patients from different backgrounds. For example, getting a parking ticket or having a car towed away may well be more stressful for working class individuals, who may lose their job if unable to get to work, than for social class I individuals, who may get a chauffeur to deal with the event while they get on with other activities. Similarly, life events – both adverse and happy – will have varying degrees of impact on individuals from different ethnic groups. A flexible and sensitive approach may well work better in eliciting the impact of a patient's experiences. If in doubt, clarify this from the family members.

WORLD VIEW

The way in which individuals make sense of the world around themselves is called 'world view', and this is very often coloured by cultural experiences and expectations as well as by past experiences and educational and socio-economic factors. Culture and ethnicity play a key role in developing a world view. In addition, group and individual identity and patients' beliefs, values and cognitive perceptions may influence their world view, which can only be ascertained by careful questioning and reading. For example, the white American view of racism and slavery may be distinctly different to that of black Americans, and the clinician, without taking sides, can produce a sense of understanding of the historical aspects of individual identity.

ACCULTURATION

As mentioned earlier, acculturation is the process whereby an individual's cultural facets may well change after coming into contact with other cultures. This process must be seen as a multidimensional phenomenon, which reflects the changes an individual goes through. Although a number of acculturation instruments are available, the best approach remains open-ended questioning covering a range of areas that are essential in understanding the process of acculturation. These are shown in Box 1.2.

It has been suggested that development of culture consciousness is a five-stage process:

1. *Naivety*: Individuals at this stage have no awareness of cultural influences on the self, and colour of the skin or ethnic and cultural identity play no role in their life.

2. *Acceptance*: This is where personal identity is defined by the 'other'. It can be passive or active acceptance, and may also create conflicts within one's self.

3. *Resistance and naming*: At this stage, individuals identify themselves as, for example, black, and its full meaning in the context of broader society is understood and may lead to anger and frustration.

4. *Redefinition and reflection*: At this stage the key task is for individuals to establish a personal consciousness in their own right.

5. *Multi-perspective internalization*: At this point individuals are able to see themselves as having, for example, a black identity with awareness in others and pride in self.

Box 1.2 Understanding acculturation

- Identify the patient's religion – its practice, frequency, rituals and taboos followed
- Identify the languages spoken – primary, where, who with, how often, degree of comfort
- Identify the patient's attitudes – towards family, marriage, cohabiting, children before marriage etc.
- Ascertain the family set-up – joint, nuclear, distance, decision making in the family
- Consider the patient's employment – degree of comfort in working with same ethnic group, work ethic, relationships
- Consider the patient's leisure activities – reading, music, hobbies, culture-related activities, language preferred
- Ascertain food preferences – religious taboos, preferred type of food, shopping
- Consider the patient's aspirations – towards self, other members of the group
- Discover whether contact is maintained or whether patient is distanced from other members of the same group

Jackson (1975) proposes that each of these five stages has an entry, adoption and exit place. Like all other processes of identity formation and development these stages can overlap with one another, and it is not essential that each stage is overcome before embarking on the next one.

The process of cultural identity and development of the self is multifaceted and complex. As discussed earlier, an interaction between migration and acculturation may occur, although not all members of minority ethnic groups are migrants or *vice versa*. The assessment of migration and its impact on individuals may become necessary in some, and is shown in Box 1.3.

Box 1.3 Assessment of migration

- Pre-migration
  - Reasons
  - Sudden/planned
  - Economic/political
  - Preparation
  - Group or individual
  - Degree of control

- Migratory
  - When did it occur?
  - Age on arrival
  - Reversibility
  - Refugee status
  - Previous similar experiences

Box 1.3 *continued*

• Post-migration	Differences between expectation and reality
	Achievement and expectation
	Attitudes towards new country
	Helpfulness of new society
	Assimilation/alienation
	Support available

MIND–BODY DUALISM

In some cultures there is no mind–body dualism perceived, and hence physical symptoms become the key idioms of distress. Some researchers have argued that psychologizers are more intelligent than somatizers, but somatic symptoms can be seen as a metaphor for underlying distress and, secondly, in view of a lack of mind–body dichotomy, such an approach is perfectly understandable. Core symptoms of depression and schizophrenia have often been reported to be universal, but when the evidence is looked at carefully, the cultural influences in presentation can be understood. The deep 'psychological reflection' common in parts of the West appears to be uncommon in other parts of the world. For example, in India there is a long history of 'inner reflection' predating Western forms by millennia, exhibiting a depth and complexity that makes the western psychology quite superficial – although it is found in theology and not always in medical traditions (Leslie and Young, 1992). In different parts of the world, internal psychological explanations of suffering are neither sought nor seen as credible (Kleinman, 1980; Shweder, 1991).

PREVIOUS EXPERIENCES

Past experiences with treatment and services may influence future help-seeking, and this in turn is bound to affect therapeutic relationships. These experiences must be explored as part of the assessment.

Basic microskills for the clinician are illustrated in Box 1.4.

Box 1.4 Basic microskills for the clinician

- Attentive listening
- Focusing
- Confrontation in a positive manner
- Following non-verbal cues
- Body language of the clinician
- Eye contact rituals
- Gaze avoidance
- Evidence of understanding

Standard mental state examination

Interested readers are referred to Goldberg (1997) for the standard mental state examination, and this will not be discussed further here. The limitations of the standard mental state examination are highlighted in this section because clinicians must be aware of the problems they are likely to face. Various cultural, social and religious groups are likely to have different and possibly unique idioms of distress.

Psychosis

Culture will often determine whether experiences of hallucinations are abnormal or not, and also whether these are understandable in a cultural context. As in developed countries, hallucinations may be seen as pathological or abnormal negative experiences; patients from other cultures may feel stigmatized and not offer information on these easily. In societies where such experiences are seen as spiritual, positive and acceptable, the patient may willingly offer information and look for affirmation of the positive experience, thereby making the clinician feel awkward (Box 1.5).

Religion and religious values influence the presentation of psychosis. As Indian, Japanese and Okinawan patients show a higher level of social withdrawal, Takeshita (1997) argues that this is an indication of the cultures from which they arrive and where religion allows withdrawal.

In both the WHO studies – International Pilot Study of Schizophrenia (IPSS) (WHO, 1974) and Determinants of Outcome of Severe Mental Disorders (DOS MED) (Jablensky, 1992) – across all centres, lack of insight was seen as the most consistent symptom. However, the same definitions of insight were used across cultures without any acknowledgement of problems of literacy, education, social class and economic standards in

Box 1.5 Examining a psychotic patient

- The interview must be in the patient's primary language

- First rank symptoms, if carefully and sensitively elicited, may give a clue to the diagnosis

- Do not make a diagnosis on a single symptom

- Be aware of cultural views and the patient's world view

- Be strict in reaching a diagnosis

- If in doubt, get a second opinion from a clinician from the same culture

- Be aware of alternative pathways into help-seeking and assess these – for example, going to a particular healer with a reputation for treating psychoses will inform you

- Evaluate each patient individually as well as a part of a culture helping the patient to understand what insight means. The clinician is better off using the emic model in identifying distress, its aetiology, expected treatments and prognosis as understood by the patient. It has been argued that African-American patients' language, behaviour and interpersonal style may be viewed as foreign, and so misunderstood that differences may be seen as evidence of thought disorder, affective disturbances and bizarre behaviour, leading to a diagnosis of schizophrenia (Jones and Gray, 1986). Epidemiological studies have been criticized by anthropologists on the basis that researchers have consistently tried to focus on similarities rather than differences.

In making sense of abnormal experiences and thoughts, the clinician must be aware of cultural nuances and factors that contribute to the contents (Box 1.6).

Box 1.6 Additional questions for abnormal phenomena

• Hallucinations	May be spiritual, positive
• Delusions	May be spiritual, positive May be negative, horrific
• Identify explanations	At individual level At cultural level
• Identify personal significance	
• Identify locus of control	

Hallucinations

These are traditionally defined as perceptions that lack sufficient basis in external stimuli, even though the patient may place their origin in the outside world. Although generally considered to be rare in normal people, they are often reported by individuals who are tired or feeling depersonalized after sleep deprivation, and very commonly after bereavement. The latter may occur for years after the bereavement experience. However, the quality of these experiences is quite different in these cases, and in some cultures have a status value. Some studies have reported religious factors and urban–rural differences in the prevalence and type of hallucinations. For example, experiences of feeling ancestors' presence and hearing their voices are related to cultural norms and cultural expectations. These experiences are often associated with concepts of the self, where individuals may perceive their existence in relation to other family or extended family members or to the village (Morris, 1994). Mukherjee et al. (1983) reported that hallucinations were more common in a sample black population than in a sample white population, and this led to the often erroneous diagnosis of schizophrenia. It is possible to differentiate between psychopathological auditory hallucinations and normal cultural variations of these experiences.

Both hallucinations and paranoid thoughts are said to be more common in smaller ethnic groups who may feel persecuted by the majority culture. Under these circumstances the patients may not wish to reveal their true mental state, and hence a repeated cautious approach without threat may prove to be successful. Stress-induced or brief, reactive psychoses must be included in the differential diagnosis. Hallucinations must be differentiated from illusions and suggestibility states.

First-rank symptoms

The two key cross-cultural studies on schizophrenia under the aegis of the World Health Organization have demonstrated that the core symptoms of schizophrenia are present across cultures and may also be seen in other conditions. However, some anthropologists have criticized these studies for focusing on similarities rather than differences (Cohen, 1992). First-rank symptoms are more likely to be picked up using the patient's primary language, and the clinicians are more likely to record these symptoms as false-positive if cultural and social factors are not taken into account.

Delusions

Delusions are often recorded as being present, but without ascertaining their cultural context. To be called a delusion, such an experience must clearly be outside the range of normal beliefs for the culture to which patients belong, and an appreciation of congruence with the patients' own culture is essential in reaching an accurate diagnosis. The clinician must understand the culture in which individuals are embedded before deciding whether the beliefs they hold are really abnormal and are pathognomonic of an underlying psychiatric disorder. The content of these beliefs is derived from the patients' cultural milieu, and is therefore most likely to be recognized as such by other members of the culture.

Delusions are said to be associated with more than 75 clinical conditions in the USA (Gaines, 1995). Given such an enormous variety and distinctiveness of ideas found across cultures, the criteria by which beliefs are perceived as abnormal are not always easy to fathom. Any beliefs that are not shared by other members of the community can be seen as incredible. Patients believe their delusions literally, and certain delusions may be more common than others – the externalization and bizarreness of these experiences must be studied carefully (Sims, 1995).

It is unreasonable to expect the therapist to have an anthropological knowledge of all the belief systems that are likely to be encountered in a multicultural practice, but the patient's family and community should provide adequate information. It is important to understand religion, cultural context and values of the patient. The clinician must put these in the formulation. If a belief is abnormal and culturally unfamiliar to members of the same community and is accompanied by functional impairment or culturally inappropriate behaviour, then it is likely to be a sign of illness.

Depression

There are several languages where no words describing depression exist. However, all cultures have words describing the sadness, tiredness, lack of energy, low mood and other symptoms that constitute the constellation of depression. Variations in the prevalence of clinical depression have been described, and Asians are said to have low rates. The reasons for this are not entirely clear; however, it is likely that, depending upon the source or data collection, the rates may differ. When a group of Punjabi women in London were interviewed, they demonstrated quite clearly that they understood the concept of depression, including its symptoms, but they were also very clear that they would seek help from religious sources such as temples and gurudwaras because depression was part of life and not a medical problem (Bhugra et al., 1997). Prevalence rates for depression have been shown to be consistently higher for women than for men across all cultures, and hence it is vital that the clinician is aware of gender roles and social expectations. As traditional beliefs about causation of depression will start to change, so will the detection rates. In traditional cultures, depression may be seen as being caused by ghost or spirit possession, or as part of life's ups and downs; the perceived external locus of control makes it very difficult to seek help, because external causes do not require internal remedies. Identifying the symptoms and then seeking help will be determined by social and cultural factors. Some cultures are more likely to present with somatic symptoms or social loneliness or alcoholism, depending upon how culture allows the symptoms to be identified and developed. Some symptoms may be universal, according to the WHO collaborative study of depressive disorders (including sadness, joylessness, hopelessness, anxiety and lack of energy), whereas other symptoms vary. In order to ascertain the presence and depth of depression, the clinicians must look out for some common features as illustrated in Box 1.7.

Bereavement can often lead to depression, but mourning and rites related to the death of an individual vary dramatically across cultures. For example, most cultures have a prescribed period of mourning interspersed with a range of rituals to allow the individuals to come to terms with their loss. The clinical symptoms of depression may be seen in bereavement, but the clinician must be aware of rituals lest a pathological grief reaction may be misdiagnosed. Thus the bereaved individual should be assessed according to the cultural norms and expectations.

Box 1.7 Key features in the assessment of depression

- Be aware of the patient's use of metaphors
- Elicit any somatic symptoms that may be metaphors for the patient's distress
- Take a detailed history of sleep, appetite and bowel disturbances, but be cautions when asking about changes in libido
- Try and understand the patient's perception of his or her distress
- Assess the patient's occupational and social norms
- Ascertain where help is being sought from
- Identity precipitants, perpetuating and predisposing factors; vulnerability factors will vary across cultures
- Place the culture in context, and do not be overwhelmed by it

Somatization

Somatization often indicates different things to different people. The soma-tizers are sometimes seen as a less sophisticated and problematic group because they do not seek appropriate psychological help. It can be argued that, by using somatization as an appropriate metaphor, these patients are using a more sophisticated approach. Somatization is seen as a trait or behav-iour that can appear in a number of clinical psychiatric conditions. Most often it is the expression of psychological distress as somatic symptoms.

Somatization has been often put forward as occurring only in less devel-oped or less industrialized societies, but this is a false perception. Somatization is common in industrialized societies such as Japan as well as in Western Europe. Tseng (1975) hypothesizes that somatization is common in China because the Chinese are exposed to Chinese traditional medicine's emphasis on the symbolic correspondence between human emotions and body organs, and also because body complaints are socially more accept-able. Two additional hypotheses suggest that the influence of media on hypochondriasis may well affect somatization and a culturally accepted reluctance to openly express sexual or aggressive findings. Similarly, for patients from the Indian subcontinent the rates of somatization are said to be higher than expected. This can be attributed to the Ayurvedic models, which do not make a mind–body distinction and hence make it likely that psycho-logical distress will be expressed in bodily form. In the same way, Chinese culture emphasizes the lack of mind–body divide, and in the Chinese lan-guage *xin jin* means 'mood' but the individual characters mean 'heart' and 'area' (or territory). Cultural differences are thus manifested more in the way the symptoms are expressed than in what patients suffer from.

Neurasthenia was a common diagnosis in Western Europe and America until the beginning of the last century, and is still used in Japan and China to describe something resembling neurotic depression. In Japan, neurasthenia has also been used as a diagnosis to hide more serious diagnoses as a result of societal stigma towards major psychoses.

Somatization can be seen in anxiety, conversion disorder, hypochondriases etc., and in more vulnerable minority ethnic groups such as refugees. Although questions have been raised regarding the overlap and distinction between hypochondriasis and somatization, it helps to make the distinction on the basis of the presence of absence of a hypochondriacal attitude and an unjustifiable anxiety.

In eliciting symptoms of anxiety, other languages will often have conceptual equivalents but not exactly equivalent words. The culturally determining factors of anxiety must be placed in the conative as well as cognitive contexts. Anxiety accompanies a large number of psychiatric disorders, and is also a separate diagnosis on its own. Acculturation has been shown to lead to reduced levels of anxiety (Shrout *et al.*, 1992), but these measurements are likely to change with subsequent generations. There are methodological problems in identifying symptoms of anxiety across cultures on a number of parameters, and the definition of the disorder itself and behaviour norms are essential prior to any surveys being carried out.

Cultural values may provide a substrate for anxiety, which then gets subsumed into somatization. Culture may also influence the manner in which anxiety symptoms manifested are then recognized as pathological in the same way that somatization is. Clinical guidelines for anxiety and somatization are illustrated in Box 1.8.

The clinician must not take culture as a synonym for unexplained variance. By talking with patients and gathering collateral information, the clinician can become sensitive to diagnostic and management issues. The

Box 1.8 Anxiety and somatization

- Recognize that anxiety is a complex substrate and somatization is a metaphor
- Anxiety and somatization may be seen as idioms of distress
- Cultural values affect anxiety and somatization
- Both anxiety and somatization may be mislabelled and misconstrued
- Both may form culture-specific syndromes
- Be aware of somatization and its causation, and anxiety and its causation; there may also be an overlap
- Be in tune with somatization and anxiety and underlying psychiatric conditions
- Be aware of underlying psychological constructs
- Be sensitive to collateral information
- Avoid cultural stereotyping and falling for easy diagnoses

symptoms of anxiety, especially if associated with panic disorder or obsessive compulsive disorder, may have religious significance in terms of purity and avoiding contamination. Some experiences may well have different cognitive meanings depending upon the culture. Culture is bound to determine the presentation of behavioural symptoms as well as affective symptoms associated with anxiety and somatization. In some cultures, the state of anxiety is viewed primarily as a collection of somatic symptoms, which may vary depending upon the culture's view of the relationship between mind and body. The clinicians must be aware of the complexities of concepts of both somatization and anxiety.

Behaviour

Some behaviours may be culturally sanctioned, such as speaking in tongues, possession states and trance states. These should be confirmed with informants and evaluated very carefully. The informant's views may well change as the behaviour changes, with or without recovery. Unusual behaviour that is not clearly understandable should not be readily seen as evidence of psychoses without due attention being paid to the adaptive or coping potential of the behaviour.

Dissociative and conversion behaviours

Conversion disorder is defined as the sudden onset of symptoms that suggest a neurological or genetic medical condition for which there is no pathophysiological explanation. All conversion symptoms could be construed as culturally sanctioned in that there are meaningful ways of expressing distress in a particular culture at a particular time, as these sanctions are dynamic and are likely to change with the passage of time. These symptoms are therefore what are seen as acceptable by the society. On the other hand, dissociative disorders are characterized by a loss of the integration of faculties or functions that are normally integrated in consciousness. This lack can influence memory, sensory modalities, motor cognitive functions and personal identity.

These conditions, and especially dissociative disorders, may be related to culturally congruent hallucinations where hallucinations are typical of the culture, even if there are true and real hallucinations. Similarly, newer concepts of falling out, indisposition, trance syndromes and possession states are included in dissociative states (Castillo, 1997). These should not automatically form the diagnosis of dissociative disorder if these experiences are not understood within the culture (see Box 1.9).

Box 1.9 Assessment issues in dissociation

- Ascertain cultural identity
- Elicit cultural explanations of both conversions and dissociation
- Ascertain cultural factors
- Ascertain social factors
- Ascertain psychological factors
- Assess cultural aspects of dyad between clinician and patient
- Do not automatically assume diagnosis
- Place symptoms in cultural context
- Negotiate clinical reality

Suicidal risk

Some cultures are more likely to have higher rates of attempted suicide. For example, women who originate from the Indian subcontinent, irrespective of their country of stay, have higher than expected rates of attempted suicide. Similarly, parent–child suicide (usually involving the mother and child) appears to be specific to Japan, Korea and China. Members of some ethnic groups (such as Indian females) who have attempted suicide are more likely to repeat the attempt. These increased rates have been linked with increased cultural turmoil (Bhugra *et al.*, 1999). Similarly, the increasing rates among European adolescents have been attributed to the growing turmoil in modern society and the loss of defined roles, particularly for men and women caught between two cultures.

The method used by suicide attempters is a direct reflection of what is easily available. In agricultural societies insecticides and pesticides are used more frequently, and where over-the-counter medications are freely available these will be used. Other culture-specific patterns of attempted suicide have been identified.

Many social and cultural factors influence patterns and attitudes towards attempted suicide. These include religion (religions that believe in reincarnation do not condemn suicide too strongly), socio-economic status (there is an inverse relationship between social class and the rates of attempted suicide), war and oppression, alcohol and drug abuse and social support (which includes family conflict).

While assessing the suicidal risk, the clinician must be aware of underlying motives and the sense of isolation, loneliness and despair, irrespective of cultural differences (Box 1.10). Planning for the attempt, suicidal intent, feelings about survival and expectations of the attempt can all guide the clinician in planning interventions. The social isolation in an

Box 1.10 Assessing suicidal risk

- Assess the suicidal risk – intent, plan, act, location, expectations
- Be aware of broad patterns of suicidal behaviour within the culture
- Explore the meaning of suicide
- Explore underlying psychiatric conditions – substance abuse, psychoses, personality disorders
- Be aware of cultural contexts of help-seeking – why here, why now?
- Distinguish between culturally sanctioned and unsanctioned suicidal behaviour

attempt or its link with an underlying psychosis make the assessment important irrespective of cultural factors.

Aggression

Cultural influences affect aggressive behaviour through culturally mediated childhood experiences. There are gender differences across cultures regarding acceptability of aggression in 150 societies (Barry *et al.*, 1976). Hostility, conflict, frustration and anger are all inter-related constructs, but aggression is behaviour whereas others are seen as emotions. Different cultures allow different ways of indulging in this behaviour, whereas emotions may be universal. Aggression is too often labelled as a manifestation of psychoses. This must be seen as cultural expression, and any assessment must be from a position of security and safety.

Violence risk and personality disorders

Risk of violence is linked with a number of psychiatric conditions, and often psychiatrists are put into the position of being custodians of individuals who may be aggressive or violent. Every culture allows a degree of violence, albeit not always formally. Culture and society will dictate how much violence is tolerated and what legal sanctions are established to deal with it. Sometimes aggressive or violent behaviour can result from psychosis and the patient's response to abnormal experiences. Other conditions such as personality disorders may play a role as well. Some cultures have been described as being generally more violent than others, but within each culture, subcultures or ethnic minority groups may demonstrate violent traits. It has been argued that homicide by black men in the USA is a kind of suicide (Hendin 1969). In addition, domestic violence in some cultures has been linked with the perception of gender roles and gender role expectations as well as with alcohol and substance misuse. Domestic violence among African-Americans has been associated with conflict due to African values, where strong women in more reciprocal relationships are faced with the macho culture learnt in the USA (Ucko, 1994).

Violence arouses strong feelings that have to be subsumed in the large cultural context. The clinician's own morality and values will play a role – both of these are culturally influenced (Box 1.11).

Box 1.11 Assessing the risk of violence

- Ascertain the various levels of aetiology of violence, including culture, biology, psychosocial factors and psychiatric conditions

- Assess the perpetrator–victim dyad

- Assess the family and developmental factors

- Be aware of subcultural values, such as gangs and migrant groups

- Ascertain the patient's acculturation and acceptance within the large group

- Be aware of your own morals, values and expectations

The term 'personality disorder' is very much culturally biased. Personality is shaped by culture and its values and norms, and pathoplasty of culture in child rearing patterns and developmental patterns must be considered in any assessment. Buffenstein (1997) argues that there are three different ways in which ethnic character can be conceptualized; ideal personality, basic personality and modal personality. The first two are clear, but the modal personality represents the most common personality type in a given community.

In order to assess the personality disorders, the clinician must learn the history of the patient's culture and subculture along with cultural identity and acculturation. Taking social occupation and personal contexts into account will allow a thorough assessment of social and personal functioning. As in psychoses, culture must not be seen as a synonym for poorly understood behaviour.

Clinical assessment across cultures must incorporate cultural sensitivity, cultural history, knowledge of cultural variations in psychopathology, and awareness of the gap between the patient and the clinician. In addition, adequate ongoing training and supervision is a must for the clinician.

Cognitive assessment

The historical and theoretical aspects of cognition and the roles of thought and language must be seen in the context of social and cultural factors. Language is very important in shaping thinking, articulation and expression. Cognitive processes may be universal, but local cultural meanings of cognitive competence will vary. The underlying theme is that cognitive functioning is related to cultural and ecological contexts – the task is to specify the general life requirements for the group as a whole and then to identify how these are communicated. The eco-cultural approach demands that such work must be accomplished prior to clinical assessment. Cultural definitions of intelligence vary across cultures, and culture-free tests must be carried out for such a purpose. The role of literacy, cognition and language must be taken into account while carrying out assessments. Similarly, processes of categorization, sorting, memory and problem solving are also affected by cultures. Standard cognitive assessments may therefore yield very little diagnostic psychopathology if used blindly across cultures. It is important to get third party information regarding memory failure and intellectual decline.

Assessment of explanatory models

In order to improve understanding, explanatory models may be used. Kleinman (1980) described these, and suggested that individuals must be asked about how they perceive episodes of sickness and treatment and how these beliefs include notions of aetiology, course of illness, meanings of symptoms, diagnosis and prognosis. Patients' perceptions of their illness underpin their interpretation of abnormal experiences and translation of these behaviours into active behaviour. The process of eliciting these explanatory models will aid the clinician to understand the patients, and allows patients to make sense of their experience (see Box 1.12).

Box 1.12 Explanatory models

- What do you call your problem/experience? What do others call it?
- What do you think caused it?
- Why do you think it has started now?
- How does it affect you?
- How does it affect others?
- What kind of problems does it cause?
- How serious do you think it is?
- Do you think it will have a long course?
- What do you fear most about your symptoms?
- Do you think it needs treatment?
- Do you think treatment will help?
- What results do you think will emerge?

Conclusions

Using the patient's models of illness may well encourage a therapist to take into account concerns of the individual while planning management. Some ethnic groups have a great respect for health professionals, such that they may not confront, question, disagree or point out the problems they are facing. This may manifest later on a selective compliance, inaccurate reporting of symptoms and consultation with other healers. Clinical needs of patients from other cultures must be addressed. The clinicians must be aware of the basic rules of cultures to which their patients belong if they are to avoid making mistakes (see Box 1.13).

Box 1.13 Good practice points

- Elicit the patient's first language, religion, ethnicity, and identification with cultural group
- Define and redefine the terms used by you and the patient to ensure understanding
- Identify idioms of distress
- Identify shared vocabulary with the patient
- Clarify the unfamiliar
- Assume nothing about the patient
- Do not be judgmental
- Be sensitive to religious and social taboos
- Communicate confidentially
- Do not use the patient's family as interpreters unless absolutely essential
- Involve carers and family as appropriate
- Discuss the findings with an independent person familiar with the culture, but within bounds of confidentiality

References

Barry, H., Josepsson L., Lauer, E. *et al.* (1976). Agents and techniques for child rearing. *Ethnology*, **16**, 191–230.

Bhugra, D., Hilwig, M., Hosein, I. *et al.* (1996). Incidence rate and one-year follow-up of first contact schizophrenia in Trinidad. *Br. J. Psychiatry*, **169**, 587–92.

Bhugra, D., Leff, J., Mallet, R. *et al.* (1997a). Incidence and outcome of schizophrenia in whites, African-Caribbeans and Asians in London. *Psychol. Med.*, **27**, 791–8.

Bhugra, D., Baldwin, D. and Desai, M. (1997b). Focus groups: implications for primary and cross-cultural psychiatry. *Primary Care Psychiatry*, **3**, 45–50.

Bhugra, D., Baldwin, D., Desai, M. and Jacob, K. S. (1999). Attempted suicide in West London II. *Psychological Medicine* **29**, 1139–47.

Brewin, C. (1980). Explaining the lower rates of psychiatric treatment among Asian immigrants to the UK. *Soc. Psych.*, **15**, 17–19.

Buffenstein, A. (1997). Personality disorders. In: M. W.-S. Tseng and J. Streltze (eds): *Culture and Psychopathology*. NY: Brunner/Mazel, pp. 190–205.

Castillo, R. J. (1997). Dissociation. In: M. W.-S. Tseng and J. Streltzer (eds): *Culture and Psychopathology*. NY: Brunner/Mazel, pp. 101–23.

Cohen, A. (1992). Prognosis for schizophrenia in the third world: a re-evaluation of cross cultural research. *Cult. Med. Psychiatry*, **16**, 53–75.

Eisenberg, L. (1977). Disease and illness: distinction between professional and popular ideas of sickness. *Cult. Med. Psychiatry*, **1**, 9–21.

Hendin, H. (1969). *Black Suicide*. NY: Basic Books.

Gaines, A. D. (1995). Culture-specific delusions: sense and nonsense in cultural context. *Psychiatr. Clin. North Am.*, **18**, 281–301.

Goldberg, D. (1997). *The Maudsley Handbook of Practical Psychiatry*. OUP.

Jablensky, A., Sartorioius N., Elnberg, G. *et al.* (1992). Schizophrenia: manifestation, incidence and course in different cultures – a WHO ten country study. *Psychological Medicine* supplement **20**.

Jackson, B. (1975). Black identity development. *J. Edu. Diversity Innovation*, **2**, 19–25.

Jacob, K. S., Bhugra, D., Lloyd, K. and Mann, A. (1998). Common mental disorders, explanatory models and consultation behaviour among Indian women living in the UK. *J. R. Soc. Med.*, **91**, 66–71.

Jones, B. and Gray, B. (1986). Problems in diagnosing schizophrenia and affective disorders among blacks. *Hospital and Community Psychiatry* **37**, 61–65.

Kleinman, A. (1980). *Patients and Healers in the Context of their Culture*. University of California Press.

Leslie, C. and Young, A. (1992). *Paths to Asian Medical Knowledge*. University of California Press.

Morris, B. (1994). *Anthropology of the Self*. Pluto Press.

Mukherjee, S., Shukla, S., Woodle, J. *et al.* (1983). Misdiagnosis of schizophrenia in bipolar patients: a multi-ethnic comparison. *Am. J. Psych.*, **140**, 1571–4.

Pederson, P. and Lefley, H. (1986). Introduction to cross cultural training. In: H. Lefley and P. Pederson (eds), *Cross-cultural Training for Mental Health Professionals*. Charles C. Thomas, pp. 5–10.

Shrout, P., Cantino, G., Bird, H. and Rubio-Stipec, M. (1992). Mental health status among Puerto-Ricans, Mexican Americans and non-Hispanic whites. *American Journal of Community Psychology* **20**, 729–53.

Shweder, R. (1991). *Thinking through Western Cultures*. Harvard University Press.

Sims, A. (1995). *Symptoms in the Mind*. Ballière Tindall.

Takeshita, J. (1997). Psychosis. In: M. W.-S. Tseng and J. Streltzer (eds), *Culture and Psychopathology*. NY: Brunner/Mazel, pp. 124–38.

Tseng, W. S. (1975). The nature of somatic complaints and psychiatric patients: the Chinese care. *Comprehensive Psychiatry* **16**, 237–45.

Ucko, L. G. (1994). Culture and violence: the interaction of Africa and America. *Sex Roles* **31**, 185–204.

WHO (1974). *International Pilot Study of Schizophrenia*. Geneva: WHO.

Principles of
management

2

Introduction

The key component in managing patients with mental illness is the thera-pist–patient interaction, which not surprisingly is influenced by a number of factors. The setting of the consultation, the age, gender and ethnicity of the therapist, as well as any past experience (especially in dealing with other cultures and socio-economic groups), along with the perceived power in the relationship, must all be taken into consideration. On the other hand, the patient's expectations, race, gender, ethnicity, models of illness, socio-economic and educational status and perceived lack of power are equally important when attempting to understand the interaction, which is also likely to influence therapeutic adherence or compliance. In order to devel-op such an adherence, the first step is for the practitioner–patient dyad to develop trust in the interaction. The clinician can influence the therapeutic effectiveness of this interaction in a number of ways. The setting in which the interaction takes place will determine the duration and acceptability of the encounter and other factors. The clinical practitioner must therefore plan the assessment and management carefully and clearly. The rationale and goals of treatment interventions must be discussed and agreed by the relevant individuals.

Mental health vs mental illness

Models of mental illness play an important role in the patients' and carers' understanding of the illness, and will therefore determine how they seek help and what their first port of call for such help is. Patients and carers are often interested in finding out why something has gone wrong, whereas clinical practitioners may be interested only in the underlying pathology. However, clinical practitioners may take into account biological, psycho-logical and social factors while trying to understand the aetiology, as well as attempting to formulate intervention strategies. Levels of disadvantage and social exclusion are not often taken into account. The idioms of distress used by the patients and their carers are very likely to be influenced by their cultures, and also by the host or majority cultures. This transition of the cultural impact depends upon the degree of contact between two cultures, the sense of belonging or alienation, the levels and degree of social support, and the appraisal of the role of mental health practitioners.

In this chapter we set out some of the key principles which health care professionals need to be aware of when planning management. Here we discuss psychological treatments whereas drug treatments are discussed in the next chapter.

Principles of management

As noted previously, the degree of contact, type of illness, type of crisis and levels of distress experienced by patients and carers, as well as unfamiliarity with the environment will all play a role in the consultation. The clinical practitioner must therefore be aware of, and indeed sensitive to, the background of the patients in terms of their culture, expectations and previous experiences. As it is very likely that, irrespective of the cultural status, the patients and their carers are have consulted other care givers, the clinical health professional should take these experiences into account while planning any interventions. As previously discussed, explanatory models (EMs) as suggested by Kleinman (1980) are a very useful concept in trying to understand patients' past experiences and their expectations of the treatment and the outcome.

The purpose of the assessment is to establish the idioms of distress and explanatory models, and to identify shared treatment goals. For patients from black and minority ethnic groups some additional information is required, and this has already been touched upon in Chapter 1. However, in some individual cases, processes of acculturation, cultural identity and racial and ethnic factors must be determined. The goals of treatment may well be broader and incorporate social interventions to a greater extent than is usual. Although well-intentioned, some interventions – especially if not indicated or if poorly timed – may well precipitate or exacerbate psychopathology. For example, when compliance becomes a focus of conflict, then not only does the therapeutic alliance break down, but also the conflict by itself (or by virtue of non-compliance) may exacerbate symptoms.

When planning treatment for black and minority ethnic groups, language, verbal and non-verbal communication and culture conflict must be taken into account. For members of these communities who are born in the UK, none or only some of these factors may be relevant. Treatment planning will be viable only with the active consent or involvement of patients and their carers, who could easily impede or accelerate the progress. When caught between two cultures, the kinship ties of a cultural group are influenced by the local customs, and with the passage of time and under these circumstances the individual clinical practitioner must steer away from preconceived stereotypes and prejudices. Careful scrutiny of local customs and cultures is required, and such knowledge will be easily accessible through the members of the patients' community. Health professionals may come from the same cultural background, but their expectations and experiences may still be remarkably different from those of the patients and their carers. The identification of patients' and their carers' idioms of distress, explanatory models and treatment expectations may not easily emerge in a single session.

Psychological treatments

Psychological treatments have been largely developed on a Euro–North American centric basis. Any provision of these services for black and minority ethnic groups brings with it its own problems of verbal and conceptual equivalence, along with the fact that some groups may find the western ego-dependent psychology as inappropriate, threatening and unacceptable in their cultural context. In those societies and cultures where the individual self remains an integral part of the society and the family, individual psychotherapy, especially if it focuses on individuation, may not be easily acceptable; and yet group work may well create more problems because the interactions in group settings may open up family secrets, thereby making it completely unacceptable on account of confidentiality. The quality of therapy offered, especially if the patients and their carers do not understand the rationale, may reduce their expectations and compliance.

One of the major problems perceived in psychotherapy is that of universalist perspective. In this context, the therapists' aim to capture the commonality between themselves and the patient where none may exist.

Definitions

Psychotherapy as a subspeciality of general psychiatry has a subset of different types of therapies – determined by the theoretical origins – where the underlying basis is that of individual change through a 'human relationship'. Such a change starts in the psychotherapy sessions and continues beyond these sessions. The types of psychotherapies are broadly divided into three categories; supportive, re-educative and reconstructive, according to Wolberg (1977). Supportive psychotherapy is for those who may be experiencing stressful life events or may have long-standing chronic illnesses where basic change is not a realistic goal. The re-educative type of psychotherapy aims to remodel the patient's thinking and behaviour by focusing on promotion and development of new and more adaptive forms of behaviour rather than on the causation. The third type of psychotherapy is reconstructive, where the primary aim is to reduce the force of irrational impulses and strivings and increase the ability to bring these impulses under control and develop a bigger range of coping strategies, both old and new. Behavioural and cognitive therapies fall into the re-educative category, whereas psychoanalytic or interpretive psychotherapies will both come into the reconstructive category. These categories are not mutually exclusive, and often a mixture of approaches may be used such as cognitive analytic therapies, cognitive behavioural therapies etc.

The universal components of psychotherapies are shown in Box 2.1.

Box 2.1 Universal elements of psychotherapy (after Tseng and McDermott, 1975)

• Basic operations	Identify and name the problem
	Prescribe remedy
	Implement
• Elements of treatment	Period of orientation
	Therapist–patient dyad
	Culturally consistent context
• Defining the cause	Dialogue
	Examination
	Genetic maps
• Explaining the problem	Comprehensibly
	Meaningfully
• Prescription for change	Change in attitude behaviour
	Ritual change

In spite of these universal components, the psychotherapies are culture-specific to some degree. For example, in addition to egocentric versus sociocentric differences, the individuals may well have to conform to 'normal' behaviour (which is identified by the society or culture at large), and these factors make the therapy culture-dependent. Not only can the therapist–patient relationship be confronting; it can also have the potential for exacerbating the patient's condition. This is more likely to occur if the patient's environmental factors are disturbed to such a degree that the relationships important to the patient are undermined (Westermeyer, 1989). Thus any psychotherapeutic intervention has to consider the wholeness of the individual and the concepts and constructs as presented to and then understood by the therapist. The expectancy of the relationship by both parties and the dependency that may result are important in understanding the interaction and the process of the relationship. In situations where the patient and therapist come from different ethnic and cultural backgrounds, the therapist who is culturally aware can move away from *a priori* assumptions and use the efficacy of adding weight to cultural factors and their significance, leading on to the development of an appropriate set of beliefs. Under these situations the therapist must be reflective and examine assumptions in power and cultural norms. The role of gender, race and ethnicity must be a part of this understanding.

The types of communication appropriate to one culture (e.g. self-disclosure, privacy, confidentiality) may not be applicable at all to another culture. A key solution offered by Bloom (1991) is to suggest that the therapist must attempt to understand how individual fantasy is transformed into interpersonal behaviour and social patterns, along with how individuals then go on to internalize, evaluate and respond emotionally to social situations and relationships. In western societies, with the 'scientific' basis of understanding, the mind is employed in delivering therapy whereas in some societies where the mind–body dichotomy is not seen as important more religio-magical therapies are followed (see Box 2.2).

Box 2.2 An example of cultural differences

Western	Eastern
Egocentric	Sociocentric
Nuclear family	Extended/joint family
Status 'achieved'	Status in the family predetermined
Weak social links	Strong social links
Choice of partner	Limited or no choice of partner
Independence	Interdependence
Individual advance	Group advance
Emphasis on newness	Emphasis on traditions

Some additional factors must be understood in their context, and these are language, racial identity and concepts of the self.

Language

The single most important component of effective communication is language. In addition to the basic exchange of ideas, interpretation and solutions, acquisition and success of language depend very much upon the socio-economic and educational status of the patient. Even in settings where both the therapist and the patient are bilingual and bicultural, one language or culture may be used more frequently than the other and one language may be employed as a defensive gesture; the therapist must be aware of this possibility. On the other hand, such switches also introduce cognitive and affective cues, which may signal a new framework of the meaning (Yamamoto *et al.*, 1993). Of course there are advantages in choosing the primary language to communicate, but the patient must decide this rather than it being a unilateral decision on the therapist's part. For example, patients with thought disorders are more easily diagnosed when interviewed in their primary language. Language plays a key role even before the interaction begins. Furthermore, in some psychotherapy services patients are asked to return a questionnaire even before the initial assessment takes place. Thus negative perceptions from the written responses of the patient on the part of the therapist, and the patient's fear of 'proper' English, may set the scene for a possible misunderstanding within the first session. In the USA, black non-standard English or other modifications of Standard English have been identified as having an effect on the therapeutic relationship. At the same time, the credibility of the therapist in the context of language usage may have important implications for engagement as well as for the therapeutic process.

When both the patient and the health practitioner share the same language and culture the therapist chooses to use this language, giving a clear message that the patient is more likely to be better understood, thereby improving the therapeutic alliance. Under these circumstances, it is important to unravel the roles of both transference and counter-transference. The role of language has not been convincingly evaluated in the outcome of therapy. The factors of transference and counter-transference are discussed later in this chapter.

As the commonality of language is not always feasible, interpreters or translators may be used and have been shown to be effective in clinical settings largely because they do not bring their own interpretations and their role is clearly understood by the basic therapeutic dyad. As time goes on in therapy, it may also be possible to switch from one language to another. Therapeutic benefits to be gained from work in the host language (or secondary language, which would generally be English) include an increasing knowledge of vocabulary and grammar on the part of the patient, learning colloquial expressions, fostering acculturation and accepting the switch to the majority language. As Westermeyer (1989) argues, it can be useful to the patient and instructive for the mental health professional to conduct therapy in both the patients' primary language and the local language if both participants have access to both languages. Both approaches have advantages and disadvantages.

Skilled interpreters can help overcome the barriers of conducting psychotherapy, provided they do not feel defensive about their culture and thus try to hide the painful or topics perceived to be shameful. Explanations for various components or types of psychotherapy may well require some comprehension of psychological concepts, and the interpreter should be able to explain or express these clearly in the patient's language. Although the presence of an interpreter can influence the dynamics of patient–health professional relationships, they are also likely to be extremely helpful if used appropriately. Westermeyer (1989) compares the relationship of the therapist and the interpreter with that of a surgeon and a theatre nurse, in that two of them can work effectively as one in achieving previously agreed goals.

Good language skills are essential for social and economic success, and language acquisition may well be one of the earliest skills required in the process of acculturation. Such a process (i.e. the acquisition of a new language) is very likely to be affected by age, social and economic factors, educational status, intelligence and linguistic ability. The patients also appear to assume languages from their therapists, depending upon the type of therapy that is being employed. The construction of reality within the therapeutic dyad is influenced by the individual's ability to use language. The therapeutic process is a fluid one, and as individuals we too go through the fluid processes of learning from others; thus the ability to speak and understand new languages will also be fluid. In some psychotherapies, for example Gestalt, the individuals are encouraged to change questions to statements in the belief that most questions are simply hidden statements about oneself. Encouraging the patient to talk in the present tense also adds power and focus to the problem, and thus a language shift is positively encouraged.

The role of language in both verbal and non-verbal communication is extremely important, and therapists must remain aware of the patient's level of linguistic knowledge in this context.

Racial and cultural identity

There is little doubt that cultural issues, especially when related to racial and cultural identity, are influential, and conflicts may well arise in the therapeutic relationship. The black and minority ethnic groups very often do not get into psychotherapy because they are seen as somatizers and not psychologically sophisticated. However, it is the poor access to services and the inability of services to address issues of culture, race and identity that appears to be a problem. Carter (1995) reports that some black patients may enter the therapeutic relationship with a number of defences related to race, such as anxiety rooted in paranoid views about the white race, which will complicate any therapeutic relationship. Although it has been argued that black therapists may be better suited to treat black patients by virtue of the fact that they have experienced discrimination and oppression, very often black therapists are trained to treat white patients with little cultural and ethnic competence. In addition, the discrimination faced by the therapists (as professionals) may well be very different, and they have often imbibed white middle-class values that may well be resented by the black patients, thereby creating more discomfort. A therapist is quite capable of misunderstanding cultural factors, and transference can be hampered by differences in cultural value orientations. The patient's race will influence the process of transference, and the patient will be influenced by the use of culture and race as an issue when in truth it may not be so. Carter (1995) proposes that although a person's level of racial identity varies, given its intricate relationship with one's world view, personality and race, the exact race-related variable is not clearly understood. The interaction can be affected by the racial and ethnic identity of the therapist and the patient, if they are of same ethnic background; and if the dyad belong to different ethnic groups, then their attitudes and beliefs with regard to their respective ethnic groups and to the 'other' will affect the therapeutic process. The interactional model is obviously important rather than race alone. Some of the key questions raised by Carter (1995) are shown in Box 2.3, and possible answers to these are shown in Box 2.4.

Box 2.3 Key questions in psychotherapy across cultures (Carter, 1995)

1. Should the therapist wait for the client to introduce the question of race?

2. How should the question of race be raised?

3. What should the therapist do if meaning of race is denied?

4. How can the therapist distinguish between racial influences and poor psychological functioning?

5. What are the ways in which race influences therapeutic interactions?

Box 2.4 Possible answers to the key questions in Box 2.3

1. Race creates the context for personality and human development; therefore race is an important aspect of one's functioning and the therapist must be trained to explore its meaning and significance

2. Success depends upon how the questions related to race are presented, therapists' training and other factors

3. Race should be seen as both a sociopolitical and psychological factor, and the therapist must be aware of this

4. Mental state functioning can be understood, along with the racial influences on it

5. Interactional dynamics are the most influenced in the therapeutic dyad

The health practitioners need appropriate training at appropriate stages, and continuing development in some of these areas. Race and racial identity are often ignored in psychotherapy, largely because organizations and institutions frequently aim to ignore it as well.

Concepts of the self

As described in Chapter 1, it is very important that the clinician understands the cultural and ethnic identity of the individual prior to undertaking any treatment. This is because such an approach allows the clinician–patient dyad not only to understand each other but also to make the strength of the (ego) identity clearer. Some psychological treatments rely on the individual's interaction with the therapist as well as the transference and countertransference. The concepts of the self can be individualistic (as in Western Europe, for example) or collectivist (as in the Eastern Europe of old). Although these are not very rigid classifications and are not always easy to define, such approaches allow the therapist to be aware of what needs to change. In individuals from sociocentric societies, if the therapist is placing too much pressure on the individual growth, such interactions may lead to a sense of failure and to complicating relationships within the family further. It is also useful to bear in mind that migrants from one kind of culture to another may or may not conform to the changes, and the sociocentric or egocentric values of the original culture may continue for one or more generations.

It is essential that the therapist is aware of the transformation of individual's fantasies to behaviour and how this behaviour is then reflected or seen to reflect onto others around the individual. Most mainstream indigenous therapies are seen in the West as systematic applications of scientific understanding of the human mind, whereas in the East, religio-magical theories dictate the development of indigenous therapies. In addition to the understanding of the concepts of the self, the value assumptions, the world view and the linguistic assumptions must be taken into account while trying to work with patients whose ethnic and cultural backgrounds are different from that of the therapist. The therapist needs to be self-reflexive and able to question his or her own assumptions about the patient, as well as the patient's assumptions about the therapist and the therapy. The types of communication appropriate for one cultural group may be completely or partially inappropriate for another group, and the changing roles within the patient's own and new cultures may add to the stress; feelings of powerlessness and rootlessness may thus need to be addressed.

Psychotherapy

The term 'psychotherapy' is often used to describe Western models of therapy. Various healing practices derived from prehistory have influenced the therapist and the development of various therapies. Anthropological and historical research has indicated that many of the concepts in modern Western psychotherapies exist in various cultures. For example, many folk tales and fairytales include notions akin to the Oedipal complex. Whatever the type of psychotherapy there are at least some common factors, including the client's motivation for psychotherapy and the fact that both components of the dyad (i.e. the therapist and the patient) have to agree to the rationale for the therapy, which then needs to be converted into a therapeutic plan. Such a therapeutic alliance must be strong enough to encourage the client to work through personal stresses and distortions, which may be ignored otherwise. Universal elements of psychotherapy are illustrated in Box 2.1.

Social, economic, educational and personal factors affect both the availability and the utilization of psychotherapy. Traditionally, psychoanalytic psychotherapy has been recommended for those who are young, intelligent, psychologically minded, articulate and well-educated. At the same time, in addition to these exclusion criteria, such therapy has not been easily available on medical insurance in the USA or on the NHS in the UK, and has thus been unable to meet the demand. In the USA, the recent emergence of encounter groups and experimental therapies can be seen as the culture's reaction against the slow, painstaking, prolonged therapy provided by psychoanalytic psychotherapy. The newer therapies are a variety of immediate, here-and-now gratification associated with the American culture. At a similar level, development of various types of behaviour therapies (especially star charts, rewards and token economy) can be seen as a mechanistic approach in a capitalist system where a malfunctioning machine is repaired without necessarily checking why it has gone wrong. Any therapy is a reflection of the culture from which it emerges. Its acceptance also very much depends upon culturally congruent metaphors for the nature of illness and the essence of healing.

Reconstructive therapies

PSYCHOANALYTIC PSYCHOTHERAPY

Psychoanalytic psychotherapy is the prime example of a reconstructive therapy. The key aim of reconstructive therapies is to cause long-term change by a reduction in the force of irrational impulses and striving to bring these under control, and increasing the range and flexibility of various forms of psychological defences. The key underlying tenet of these therapies is the premise that the individual's personality is dynamic in its constitution, and various types of experiences affect the individual's growth and produce impulses and desires that lead to conflicts between the individual's system of ideals, values and standards, and reality. Repression of these feelings and reactions affects the individual's functioning. In order to carry out such therapies, the therapist is required to have special training, personal psychoanalysis and supervision.

Freudian psychoanalytic psychotherapy is an extensive as well as an intensive form of exploratory psychotherapy. The three key concepts of psychoanalysis are free association, interpretation and transference. The intense nature of the relationship between the therapist and the patient in the form of transference allows the therapist to explore various relationships the patient has been through and to work towards termination. Jungian psychoanalytic psychotherapy, on the other hand, emphasizes the value of patients pursuing the products of unconscious fantasy through dreams, reveries and artistic creativity, the role of archetypes and individualization through the emphasis of spiritual factors. The underlying functions of psychoanalytic therapy emphasize individual functioning. These therapies, therefore, reflect the culture-specificity of the milieu in which they were developed and are practised. Therefore, universal applicability cannot be taken for granted. The field has been extensively reviewed by the feminist and cultural overviews which suggest, for example, that male white therapists should understand their own feelings, and the detrimental effects of their guilt and need for being all-powerful.

The phenomena of transference and counter-transference in mixed ethnic cultural settings indicate that an additional set of factors may be at play. The core religious or spiritual values may play a more important role in identity development, as does the sociocentrism or the egocentrism. The role of the Oedipal complex in non-nuclear families must be understood by therapists. The linking of defence mechanisms and sexual thoughts with religion and moral values changes the perceptions of both the therapist and the patient.

BRIEF DYNAMIC PSYCHOTHERAPY

This type of psychotherapy involves a short, intense form of treatment (generally between 10 and 40 sessions, but more often between 10 and 20 sessions) specifically targeting problems by the confrontation of pathological defences and transference. The basic aim of such an approach is to build a strong therapeutic alliance and help the patient resolve a specific intrapsychic conflict. There are different approaches, such as cognitive analytic therapy, which will require extensive training, and the therapist has to enable the patient to confront defences, and interpret transference, resistance and counter-transference. Underlying motivational strength and an ability to trust the therapist, along with capacity to lead on to termination of the therapy without undue emotional trauma, are critical in tolerating and dealing with the anxiety provoked by such therapies. Such therapeutic approaches have to be based on the depth of rapport, the nature of hidden feelings, the degree of anxiety and pain, and the way in which the patients deal with these.

Such a therapeutic approach differs from the focused supportive therapy described below. Under certain circumstances, brief, dynamic psychotherapy is more appropriate for clients from other cultures. However, as with psychoanalytic psychotherapy, the understanding of transference resistance, dream analysis and the analysis of defence mechanisms are likely to vary across different cultural and ethnic groups. The mixture of such an approach with cognitive and behavioural therapies is more acceptable for patients from other cultures.

GROUP THERAPY

It is argued that the underlying dynamics within a group act as a model to encourage the individual to develop greater self-awareness, sensitivity and social skills. The group may be classified according to the theoretical orientation of the therapists, the composition of the group (number of people, their age, sex and cultural background), the timing and number of sessions, and the specific aim of the group. The group must work together to reach an element of cohesion and trust, and allow individuals to identify and go on to accomplish specific group tasks.

It could be argued that groups can be used more successfully with cultural and ethnic groups that have a more sociocentric bent. However, the notions of shame and dishonour may become a block to active participation. By using a mixture of approaches, these problems can easily be overcome.

Re-educative psychotherapies

In some ways re-educative psychotherapies could be the most appropriate type to bring about relevant changes, provided these are not seen as dictatorial or culturally demeaning by the patients and their carers. When used carefully, such approaches can prove to be culturally appropriate and acceptable and also extremely successful. These therapies include behaviour, cognitive and humanistic therapies. The chief aim is readjustment, the modification of goals and the relearning of habits and attitudes, without necessarily focusing on or changing the insight. As the individual becomes trained to change maladaptive patterns of adjustment, a sense of self-mastery and an increase in self-esteem emerges, leading to better functioning.

BEHAVIOUR THERAPY

When an observable behaviour is unacceptable to the patient or their carers, behaviour therapy can be especially useful. As culture and society frequently determine which behaviour is acceptable and which should be seen as deviant, such therapies can be seen as more appropriate if they are not seen as imposing and punitive. Working with black and minority ethnic groups, behaviour therapies have been shown to have mixed results – while some studies have shown excellent results (Turner, 1982), others have not done so (Bhugra and Cordle, 1986, 1987). However, with appropriate modifications (i.e. by changing the structure or adding psychoanalytic interpretations), outcome can be improved (d'Ardenne, 1986; Gupta et al., 1989).

In sexual dysfunction, especially where the purpose of sexual intercourse is seen as procreative and not necessarily as a pleasurable activity, it is likely that sensate or genital focusing may not be seen as an appropriate intervention, especially if the couple live in a joint family setting or do not have enough privacy. Similarly, social skills training, assertiveness training or even anger management may be seen as inappropriate interventions if the patients and their carers are not involved in decision-making and these are against the society's mores. The emphasis on dating when that is not the accepted form of meeting members of the opposite sex, and social skills focused on such an approach, can produce major discord between the therapist and the patient. The way forward is to establish a clear set of norms, which are then negotiated with the patients and their carers so that a broadly similar set of expectations is modified as the therapy progresses.

The functional analysis of behaviour therapy takes place in seven steps, and these are shown in Box 2.5. Of these, social relationships and the norms of the patients' environment are most likely to be influenced by social and cultural norms.

For behaviour therapy, relaxation techniques are often the first step, along with education. Of course other relaxation techniques like yoga and meditation can be used, but the therapist must be aware that not all individuals originating from the Indian subcontinent will follow or be interested in such approaches. A modification of strategies to suit individual needs must be the essential first step.

Like relaxation techniques, modelling is often used to help patient acquire new behaviours by imitation. Here too, results of the intervention are said to be better if the patients are able to identify with the person serving as the model. Another way forward is for the therapist to work closely with family members, who can become part of the therapy through being co-opted as co-therapists.

With other forms of behaviour therapy, such as biofeedback for pain management, the individual patients and their relatives must be involved in assessment and management.

Box 2.5 The seven steps of functional analysis

1. Clarification of the problem

2. Understanding of the function of the problem

3. Motivation

4. Developmental analysis

5. Self-control

6. Social relations

7. The patient's environment

COGNITIVE AND BEHAVIOUR THERAPY

Cognitive and behaviour therapy is being used increasingly in Asia. Psychotherapy was almost unheard of in non-Western settings until after the Second World War, and even now its acceptance and progress has been limited. Its increased use can be attributed to the impact of British rule, overseas aid and other closer ties with cultures where psychotherapy is available and used. As noted earlier, such an import is often carried out without any clear indication for its usage; there is blind acceptance because psychotherapy is a science, and all science is universal. Behaviour therapy and cognitive therapy are good examples of Western psychological techniques being imported unquestioned into non-Western settings without a proper examination of the validity and utility in the new environment. It is now understood that the development of behaviour and cognitive therapies is dependent upon a number of cultural, social, economic, political and technological factors. Culture and ethnicity have often not been explicitly acknowledged as explanatory variables in the functional analysis of behaviour (for further discussion, see Oei and Goh, 1998). As these authors argue, going to a therapist – a stranger in the eyes of patients and their carers – is in itself a social taboo, largely because this is an acknowledgement of the fact that a family member is having emotional problems or psychological difficulties will reflect badly and bring shame and dishonour to the family name. As mentioned earlier, the sociocentrism or collective nature of the family in certain cultures makes it likely that the therapist is seen in a hierarchically powerful position, and the interactive nature of behavioural and cognitive therapies makes it difficult to be accepted. As these therapies are influenced by the Western models, the underlying ideologies and values play an important role in influencing interactions. Singh and Khan (1998) have highlighted some of the key problems in using behavioural therapy in developing countries. Of these the first is religion, in that religious beliefs often act as taboo; they found that a patient found it difficult to use sexual imagery for orgasmic reconditioning. They suggest that this can be overcome, as has been shown in India where stories from the scriptures can be used to overcome some of the problems. Singh and Khan (1998) illustrate this by citing a case where the patient was suffering from a continuing doubt that he might have uttered the word 'divorce' three times thereby turning his ongoing marriage into adultery or extramarital sexual sin. The authors asked a religious preacher to tell him that even if he did so, his marriage was still legal, and thus helped him overcome this. Similarly, using concepts of external locus of control allows the therapist to be part of the externality to help the patients overcome some of the problems. Another problem highlighted by these authors is the role of superstitions in cultures. The rules of disclosure and somatic expression are two additional factors of which the therapists must be aware. A key problem, as mentioned in Chapter 1, is that by applying strict Western criteria for diagnosis, often the disclosure of emotion does not fit into standardized categories. There is every likelihood that disclosures of somatic and psychological states may thus differ in form as well as content. It is only by being aware of cultural subtleties and nuances that the clinicians can reach a diagnosis that allows them to make appropriate interventions. Wooding and Oei (1998) suggest that for Australian aboriginal people, factors such as loss of lands, culture, discrimination, alienation from the rest of the society, poor socio-economic status and poor housing all contribute to what has been called social depression. However, Coaby (1991) emphasizes that if every case of depression in this group is attributed to social factors, then those whose depression can be treated individually may feel cheated.

A blind application of cognitive and behaviour therapies is doomed to failure. The clinicians must be aware of the advantages and disadvantages of each modality, and must modify their approaches accordingly.

COGNITIVE THERAPY

Like behaviour therapy, cognitive therapy is problem-oriented and aimed at correcting cognitive schema, which then allow patients to improve their coping skills and strategies. The aim of the therapy is to change the negative cognitions and enable the patient to develop appropriate intervention strategies. Such an approach relies on information processing as the basis of a therapeutic effect. It is time-limited and structured, and the therapeutic intervention follows a clear structure. Such an approach means that the patient, in conjunction with the therapist and in a structured way, identifies the tasks that have to be carried out between therapy sessions. A rationale for the problem management is offered, which can then be used as part of the training for problem management and problem solving. The patients are trained to overcome their distress and taught future coping strategies. The basic components of cognitive therapy are illustrated in Box 2.6.

The basic aim of cognitive therapy is to encourage patients to monitor their negative automatic thoughts and to encourage them to understand the links between cognitions, affect and behaviour. The cognitive triad of depression – negative thoughts about self, future and the world – has not been studied or evaluated in other cultures and ethnic groups. It is obvious that concepts of self and the resulting guilt or shame will differ across cultures, thereby making an automatic application of the triad improbable if not entirely impossible. Basic underlying theoretical assumptions must be studied to establish underlying norms. The usefulness of cognitive therapy has been established in various clinical settings, and will allow further application if the theoretical basis is understood. It is no doubt cheap, time-limited and focused, and the patients, as in psychoanalytic psychotherapies, do not have to be introspective or verbally expressive.

Box 2.6 Components of cognitive therapy

- Define the problem clearly
- Identify the objective factors
- Identify factors for vulnerability
- Identify mediational cognitive factors
- Identify coping skills
- Identify current themes
- Identify emotional factors
- Set achievable tasks
- Evaluate achievements and set new tasks
- Teach coping strategies

HUMANISTIC PSYCHOTHERAPY

Client-centred psychotherapy highlights those aspects of the patient's functioning that follow the process of self-actualization. The emphasis results from the therapist's unconditional positive regard, empathy and genuineness, which enable the patient to work with the therapist.

Walsh and Vaughan (1980) suggest that four dimensions of consciousness, conditioning, personality and identification in a transpersonal approach are the cornerstones of humanistic therapies. This model includes a spiritual domain as well, thereby making it more attractive for some ethnic minority groups. However, much work needs to be done in establishing the use of and evaluation of such therapies across different cultural settings and in different ethnic groups.

Supportive psychotherapies

Such therapies include occupational therapy, music therapy, reassurance, ventilation, guidance and milieu therapy, depending upon patients' clinical conditions and needs. The objectives of such therapies are: to minimize the impact of an impending threatening event; to provide protection and relief from responsibility during transitional periods; and to encourage expression of feelings along with talking through various theoretical and practical difficulties. Such an approach is not suitable for change, but enables the individual to cope with chronic and disabling conditions. However, such an approach is extremely useful when the individual is stressed due to long-term problems, or is undergoing psychosocial transitions.

Supportive psychotherapies can be used for helping individuals to build up their skills to a point where more profound, time-consuming and complex interactive psychotherapeutic interventions can be employed for long-term changes. The key components of psychotherapy include interview (which is the most important point in the contact, as discussed earlier), reassurance, explanation, guidance suggestion and ventilation. Bland reassurances without an understanding of cultural and social expectations mean that any attempt towards working together is likely to fail miserably. In cultures and societies where interdependence is encouraged and is essential for survival, the purpose of therapy has to be modified accordingly. Under these circumstances, attempts to provide direction towards independence and individuation are not only doomed to failure but will also produce a strong feeling of ambivalence and cultural confusion in the minds of the patients and their carers, and a cultural fog in the mind of the therapist.

Similarly, occupational or music therapy may not be of any interest to the patients or their carers because it does not meet with their expectations, simply because the purpose of music may be seen as dramatically different when compared across cultures. Occupational therapy may be seen as too trivial and beneath the dignity of the individual, and may be seen as intrusive if emphasis is on teaching cooking skills to males in cultures where gender roles do not allow them to cook (for detailed discussion, see MacCarthy, 1998).

Other therapies

Other therapies include couple and marital therapy, family therapy and indigenous therapies.

COUPLE AND MARITAL THERAPY

Couple and marital therapy emerged from clinical observations that the relationships between the couple can elucidate individual psychodynamics and facilitate psychotherapeutic interventions. Theoretically, the systems approach has been used in development of various forms of therapy (see Crowe and Ridley, 1990). This involves an awareness of the role of marriage and its influence on the functioning of individuals in the relationship and the couple as a unit.

When working with a couple where both members belong to the same culture but a different one than that of the therapist, the latter must be aware of the role of marriage and sex within their culture. The role of the therapist could be that of a village elder, providing advice, support and guidance. In some societies, for example, marriages are arranged between families and hence the families 'marry' families rather than individuals marrying individuals. The style and content of marital therapy will therefore have to reflect this.

If the two members of the couple belong to different cultures themselves, additional factors come into play. Under these circumstances, the approach will have to be different. The members of the couple and the therapist may come from different ethnic and cultural backgrounds, which may affect their expectations for help-seeking and help provision respectively. A key factor in the therapist–client interaction is the understanding of the problems and managing a strategy, which allows the two sides to work together towards the same goal. In addition, while projecting such an interaction, mutual expectations and past expectations tend to play an important role (see Figure 2.1).

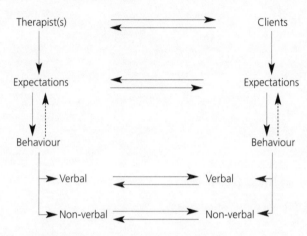

Figure 2.1   The therapeutic encounter.

As already noted, it can be argued that psychotherapy or therapy of any kind is culture-specific and also Eurocentric. However, within each mode of psychotherapy there exist key elements that can be seen as universal. These are the basic operations of identifying and naming problems, and prescribing remedies. A second component is that of the elements of treatment, which includes the period of orientation, establishing a therapeutic relationship and the 'theatre' of the management. Defining the causes of the problem through dialogue, dreams and examinations, and explaining the problem through meaningful and comprehensible understanding, can then be used to lead on to recommending prescriptions for change.

The cultural context of such an interaction is discussed at length later, but will bring with it the microcosm of the society and the inherent power in the therapist–client interaction, which is affected by bigger factors that affect the society at large.

Couples and therapists

The interaction between the therapist and the clients can be affected in a number of ways (see Figure 2.2). Within such an interaction there are several scenarios, all of which have implications for the planning of management:

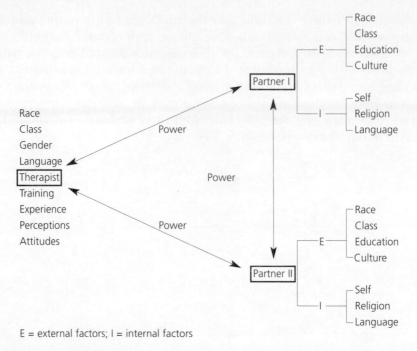

E = external factors; I = internal factors

Figure 2.2 Therapeutic relationships.

1. The therapist may come from the majority culture and the couple from the minority culture.

2. The therapist may come from the minority culture and the couple from the majority culture.

3. The therapist may be from the majority culture, whilst one of the partners is from the majority culture and the second from a minority culture.

4. The therapist may be from the minority culture, whilst one of the partners is from the majority culture and the second from a minority culture.

5. The therapist may belong to mixed race category, as could one or both of the partners (see also Figure 2.4).

Each of these dyads – taking the couple as one 'unit' – will have a set of expectations and problems that need to be considered by the individual therapist while planning any interventions. Within such a dyad, three key components must be emphasized. These are, first, the ethnocentrism of the couple, the therapist and the culture surrounding such a dyad. Secondly, within the dyad interaction there will be an imbalance of power related to communication (both verbal and non-verbal) and experiences of oppression. The third component is alliance, where the therapist and the couple forge an alliance to more forward, and such an alliance comes from the disorder itself and the shared world view.

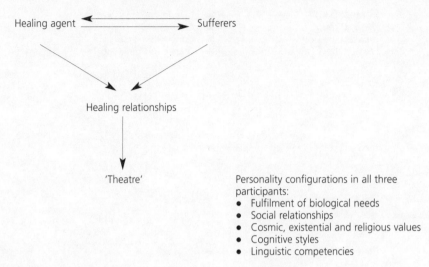

Figure 2.3   Interactions between the couple and the therapist.

The healing relationship functions in the 'theatre', but has personality and social configurations as an integral part. These are illustrated in Figure 2.3. The relationship between the therapist and the clients depends upon personality configurations and fulfilment of biological needs, along with other internal values such as cosmic, existential and religious values, and external factors such as social relationships and the type of society the couples come from and live in. The power relationship between the therapist and the two partners is a microcosm of the society; the power has been given to the therapist by virtue of professional experience and the role he or she plays in the interactions. As noted earlier, the past experience of the therapist and the patient may influence interactions in such a way as to make therapeutic progress difficult. This is further complicated in the setting of couple therapy, where two individuals each with their separate expectations, roles and power relationships present for therapy. If the members of the couple are from the same cultural background, then the interactions between the couple and therapist may raise different issues to when all three members come from different ethnic and cultural backgrounds. These various settings are shown in Figure 2.4.

Key issues regarding mixed race relationship couples and therapists are highlighted in Box 2.7.

Depending upon the culture and society from which the couple come, the notions of self and the importance of sociocentrism will both play a significant role not only in the relationship but also in help-seeking as well as in acceptance of any therapeutic interventions. The individual's notions of self and self-esteem are equally important. Cross-cultural definitions of family may well differ, and although some couples may be in nuclear set ups, these may be a collaboration that functions as an extended or joint

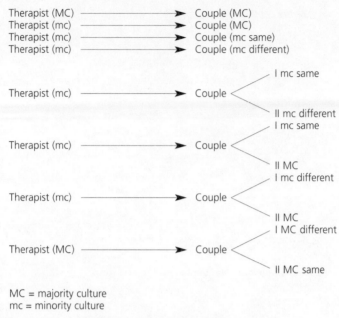

MC = majority culture
mc = minority culture

Figure 2.4   Various settings of couple and therapist interaction.

family. On the other hand, within extended or joint living arrangements the couple may have separate cooking arrangements, thereby making 'individuation as a couple' possible. Theoretically, the systems approach is the most appropriate assessment and management strategy, and this can also work in a culture-free environment. The style and the content of assessment and management have to reflect appropriate components of the culture.

Box 2.7 Key stages in the couple–therapist relationship

• Assessment	Problem
	Couple
	Culture
• Engagement	Couple
• Therapeutic relationships	Transference
	Counter-transference
	Directive/non-directive
• Termination	Transference
	Counter-transference
	Cultural factors

Couple therapy may not be easily accepted by various cultural and ethnic groups, and the therapist must recognize that in some situations it is not the couple but the whole family that may be the 'target' for the therapeutic intervention. The key aim is to try to be aware of one's own strengths and weaknesses, including a lack of knowledge.

Assessment

In the early stages of referral and assessment, therapists must be aware of their own feelings and expectations (see Box 2.8). The assessment in

Box 2.8 Therapist's self-examination

- Be aware of own likes, dislikes, stereotypes, racism, lack of respect
- Be aware of own identity – ethnic, cultural, concepts of self, gender, sense of power
- Be aware that mutual learning is possible
- Be aware of a tendency to idealize one or other culture
- Be aware of the strengths and weaknesses of own culture as well as other cultures

psychotherapy in general and couple therapy in particular relies on a number of factors, which are shown in Figure 2.5, and in Boxes 2.9 and 2.10.

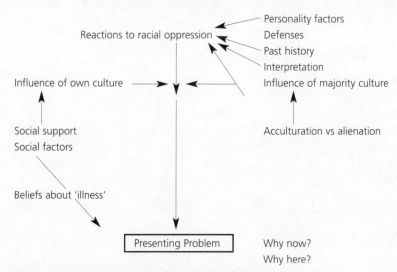

Figure 2.5   Presenting problems and antecedent factors

Box 2.9 Assessment in couple therapy

- Racial/ethnic similarities
- Racial/ethnic differences
- Race may/not be an issue
- Religious beliefs/taboos
- Meanings attached to therapy
- Meanings attached to the role of therapy
- Definitions of family
- Role of couple *vis a vis* family
- Family's expectations of the couple
- Feedback on what is wrong and what is right
- Use of translators/interpreters
- Clarify the problem
- Clarify the definition of the problem
- Clarify concepts of self
- Clarify cultural identity
- Establish choice of therapeutic modality
- Establish hypotheses and workability

Box 2.10 Assessment in couple therapy

• Clarify terms	
• Identify problem	How defined? Who defined? Why now? Why here?
• Cultural norms	
• Expectations	Of each other Of therapy Of therapist
• Roles in relationship	Financial Decision making Children Level of intimacy Household responsibility

Box 2.10 *continued*

- External sources of stress
- Strengths of relationship
- Bicultural existence
- Remarriage/fidelity

Cultural norms for the couples must be assessed (see Box 2.11), and this assessment includes questions about norms for the marriage and expected roles and responsibilities within the relationship.

Box 2.11 Assessment of cultural norms

- Normative age for marriage?
- Why at that age?
- Do men have to achieve certain things prior to getting married?
- When are men/women considered eligible for marriage?
- How much free will do they have to get married?
- History of arranged marriage?
- Definition of arranged marriage?
- Whose responsibility?
- Do these patterns continue with migration?
- Other basis for mate selection?
- If different, how so?
- How is it accepted by the culture?
- Role of common interest, mutual attraction, love or lust?
- Expected duties of husband/wife?
- Gender roles?
- Division of responsibilities?
- Power? Alteration of power equation?

The assessment for couple therapy generally focuses on the quality of the relationship, because that is where the problem is based. However, additional problems such as sexual dysfunction may underlie the relationship difficulties, so the therapist must be aware and sensitive in order to elicit sexual problems that may indeed be the primary cause of relationship dysfunction. The therapist must be able to ascertain the quality and the strengths and weaknesses of the relationship, so that appropriate interventions can be put in place. It is imperative that assessment is value-free and culturally sensitive so that management can occur. In interracial unions, the strength of relationship may result from factors such as more thorough preparations for marriage and greater commitment to the relationship (see Box 2.12).

Box 2.12 Inter-ethnic marriages/relationships

Advantages	Disadvantages
More thorough preparation for marriage	Probably less rigidity in relationships
Greater degree of commitment	Possible isolation
Greater degree of self–other-differentiation, tolerance, respect, acceptance	Sense of loss of self
	Social stigma
Broader opportunities for learning growth	Institutional racism
Greater opportunities for children	
More accepting of differences	

In the early stages of assessment, the therapist should be aware of the reasons for referral and the expectations of therapy.

Possible pitfalls

Some of the key problems in psychotherapy in general, and couple therapy in particular, are related to issues like missionary racism. This is where clinicians rather patronizingly convey to patients that their role and goal is to 'save them from their plight' or to take care of these 'poor' people who are unable to look after themselves, and end up either being too controlling or too closely identifying with the patient. In couple therapy such a problem is further compounded, so that if therapists are not aware of their feelings towards race and ethnicity they may over-identify with one person and become too controlling towards the other. Some of the possible pitfalls are illustrated in Box 2.13.

Box 2.13 Dangerous assumptions and responses on part of the therapist (after Ridley, 1995)

Colour blindness	Assumption that minority client is the same as majority client
Colour consciousness	All problems result from the minority status
Cultural transference	Patients' feelings result from therapists' race
Cultural counter-transference	Therapists' feelings towards patients result from their own race
Cultural identification	Minority therapists over-identify everything in terms of racism and define problems as racially based
Identification with oppressor	Minority therapists deny their status by virtue of power and because it is painful

In addition, due to cultural and ethnic factors, individual patients or therapists can be seen as dominant whether they come from the majority culture or not. The advantages and disadvantages for therapists of the various dyad interactions are shown in Box 2.14.

Box 2.14 Advantages and disadvantages of dyads

	Advantages	Disadvantages
MC therapist/MC patient	Reaffirm culture, shared identity and experiences	Lost opportunity to grow/ learn more about patients
MC therapist/mc patient	Awareness of differences	Sense of cultural inequality and communication
mc therapist/mc patient	Shared identity and experiences, credibility	Loss of hope, possible lack of confidence
mc therapist/MC patient	Shared learning	Poor communication

MC = majority culture
mc = minority community

Strategies

Two key strategies in the therapeutic intervention are educational and psychological. As illustrated in Box 2.15, these approaches suggest that the therapist is primarily an educator with both educative and psychological

Box 2.15 Educational/psychological strategies

Understanding social and cultural differences	Educational strategy
Coping with peers and majority culture	Psychological strategy
Communicate effectively	Educational/psychological strategy
Acquire social skills	Psychological strategy
Acquire language	Educational strategy
Coping with stress	Psychological/educational strategy
Psychology of minority cultures	Psychological strategy
Concepts of self	Educational/psychological strategy

functions. These strategies are not mutually exclusive, and should be used in conjunction with other therapeutic approaches.

In some situations, the members of minority ethnic groups may bring with them indigenous therapies and use these along with psychotherapy and pharmacotherapy. These are discussed in detail in Chapter 3. Suffice it to say that some therapies developed in cultures from which individuals emerge may be used in other settings as well (see Lloyd and Bhugra, 1993; Bhugra and Bhui, 1998). Combining different types of therapies is not necessarily contraindicated, but therapists must be aware that not enough evaluation research data are available.

As MacCarthy (1988) points out, cognitive therapy often relies on prescribing 'healthy' ways of thinking and moral authority is vested in the beliefs and values of the therapist and passed on to the patient through a system of rhetoric (Totman, 1982). She argues that the affective impact of many cognitions partly depends upon the set of beliefs and norms shared by a salient social group. Some of the healthy thoughts 'prescribed' by cognitive therapists may be congruent with the values and experiences of middle-class whites in the West, but may well clash with the world views and practical and economic experiences of limited choice and alienation. The struggle for personal control versus external locus of control can create difficulties for individuals and therapists.

Family therapy

MacCarthy (1988) argues very cogently that structures which signal health in Western nuclear families may not accurately reflect the underlying situation where enmeshment may be seen as pathological. As the form and content of roles of families vary widely across cultures and societies, it is only appropriate that assessment and management take these into account (Box 2.16). In addition to sociocentric values, mutual dependence,

Box 2.16 Steps for assessing family factors

- Understand the family structure – genograms may help
- Understand the normative structures in the community
- Identify the 'gender' and other roles
- Identify the role expectations
- Identify the conflict between role and expectations
- Identify levels of acculturation in all those who will form a part of the 'family session'
- Identify the world view and language competence

loyalty and obligation may be expected, and any attempt on the therapist's part to modify these is likely to run into resistance and social isolation on the part of the individual/couple.

In some cultures extended family may be the norm even if this is not through the marriage line but through strong kinship networks and adaptability, which determine the family support. Another complication highlighted by MacCarthy (1988) is the altered roles and role expectations within the family. She cites the 'parental child', as seen in black American and African-Caribbean families, as an example. In addition, the therapist must be aware that family constellations and structures are not necessarily static and will evolve and change in response to altered contacts with majority culture as part of the process of acculturation.

When a family therapist is faced with an unfamiliar cultural and family setting, the first step is to identify what in the family context is being seen as dysfunctional. Adequate information needs to be obtained to ascertain these definitions. In the identified patient scapegoating can easily occur, and the therapist must be sensitive about the symbolic value of the symptom and how this can be incorporated into the treatment strategy.

Generational conflict is relatively common, but its role in black and minority ethnic groups is often not clear. Younger generations, as part of their acculturative process, may see themselves as part of the majority culture, and may wish to move away from the 'traditional' culture – where role expectations are quite different. Such conflict may involve the therapist as well, who may see things from a majority or establishment perspective. In addition to identifying the relative structures of the family, therapists must be aware of the stigma that may shroud the family, which is seen to be 'washing its dirty linen in public'. The role of the social services, legal system and child care and adoption agencies must be seen in this context.

In any therapeutic interaction between the Western-method oriented and trained family therapist and the minority family, areas of symbolic meaning must be considered, especially in personal meanings such as family structure and language as well as in communication. The role of cultural meanings in symptoms should be clearly understood in order to make sense of their experiences and communications so that appropriate interventions can be placed in context. Differences in family structures and organization relate not only to authority and establishment, but also to continuity and interdependence with family and kinship ties. If it is likely that feelings and emotions are not expressed openly, clearly and directly, the therapist may have to resort to using indirect means with shared symbols. External factors that are also likely to be related to larger society, such as racism, poverty and poor educational opportunities, may also contribute to a sense of alienation, and the therapist must be able to understand this. Even if, practically, the therapist is unable to do anything, an open and honest acknowledgement of material disadvantage and other external factors will establish an openness and honesty in the interaction. A perceived lack of power and a sense of frustration may undermine the therapeutic task (see Figures 2.6 and 2.7).

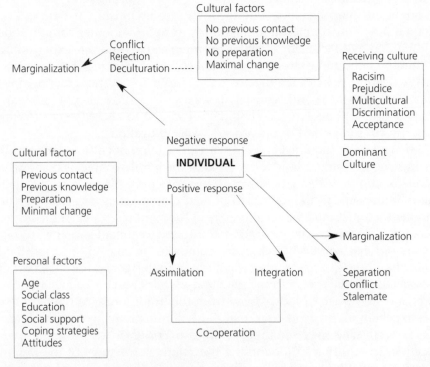

Figure 2.6 Association of cultural and psychological impacts.

In therapy, the therapist and the family should at an early stage be aware of the purpose of the therapy and agree to mutually set goals. These could be goals related to situational stress (such as social isolation), goals related to dysfunctional patterns of cultural transition and goals related to

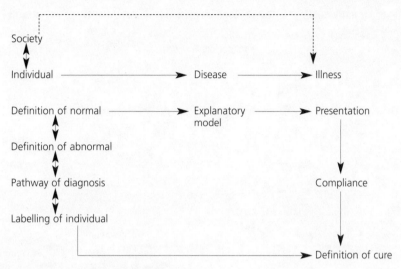

Figure 2.7   Society–illness interaction.

cross-cultural dysfunctional patterns. The majority society generally expects the minority groups to fit in with the majority. Such a process in which mutually agreed goals are set is based on the assumption that the therapist will adhere to the value orientation of a specific minority family. Individual psychologically oriented goals are not likely to fit in with the emphasis on families and interdependence. Intergenerational factors, parent–child relationships and sibling relationships all have different meanings across different cultures. If the family structure is extended, then the family therapy sessions need to recognize the fact and also involve relevant people either on a regular basis or, more practically, on a 'when required' basis.

Following on from the mutually agreed goal setting, the therapist should recognize the focus and the system unit for therapy. Understanding and respecting the ethnic minority family's cultural norms and present social context are perhaps the most important skills in selecting a subsystem unit for therapy. The family's need for privacy on one hand and the hierarchical and vertical nature of families in some cultures on the other, along with extended families, indicate that the therapist must remain sensitive and aware at all times. Working separately with subsystems in the family and then bringing them together will confirm to the family that the therapist is aware of the subsystems. Using such an approach also means that the therapist can allow different members of the family to express their true thoughts and negative feelings. Acculturation and self-esteem go hand in hand (see Figure 2.8). Depending upon different therapeutic orientations of the therapists, different approaches can be used. Ho (1987), for example, recommends a 12-techniques-and-skills approach for problem solving. The key goals include resolution of situational stress, cultural transitional

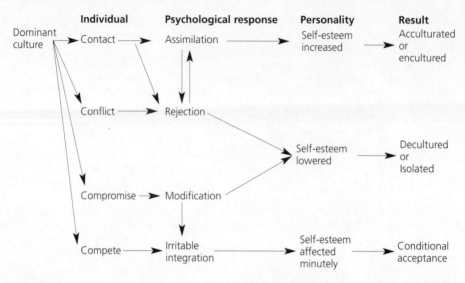

Figure 2.8   Hypothetical model of relationship between acculturation and self-esteem.

conflicts and, lastly, conflicts within the family. For resolving situational stress, the therapist should try and mobilize and restructure the extended family network. As minority ethnic groups often use pluralist systems of managing problems, working closely with other healers may demonstrate a degree of openness on the part of the therapist and also make it possible to bring in a co-therapist. Using domiciliary assessments and employing role and model techniques and the advocate role allows the therapist to work closely with the family, especially to reduce the situational stress. In order to deal with cultural transitional conflicts, the therapist can work with the family by remaining fair and firm without taking sides but being willing to look at the conflict from both sides and find a commonly acceptable ground.

While attempting to resolve family and relationship problems the therapist must be aware of his/her own feelings and self-reflection, as indicated in Box 2.8. The therapist can follow the team, team leader or wise man approach, or be a therapist-helper.

Family therapy is summarized in Boxes 2.17–2.26.

Box 2.17 Psychiatric patients and the role of family members

- Providers of information
- Recipients of information
- Co-operators of treatment
- Saboteurs of treatment
- Helped by the treatment of the patient
- Made worse by the treatment of the patient
- Cause of disorder
- Central focus for intervention

Box 2.18 Presentations of family

- Marital issues may be reflected by the children
- Disturbances may affect marriage
- Psychosexual difficulties
- May precipitate serious mental illness
- Childhood disorders

Box 2.19 Indications for family therapy

- Agreement that there is a problem requiring resolution
- Willingness to commit themselves to attend
- Commitment that the family will stay together
- The problem may be of individuation
- Scapegoating is out of cultural context
- The family is willing to participate actively, though this may vary culturally

Box 2.20 Criteria affecting the achievement of goals in family therapy

- Cultural, class, occupational and educational background
- Perceptions and experiences of marriage and family
- The relationships between family members
- Personality development – individual and cultural factors
- Duration, circumstances and cultural expectations of the marriage

Box 2.21 Conceptual framework for family work with ethnic minority families

Check:
- Reality for the group (e.g. racism, poverty, education)
- Biculturation
- Ethnic differences in minority status, and migratory experience
- Ethnicity and external factors – collective vs individual social class
- Ethnicity and internal factors – language, self-esteem.

Box 2.22 Preparation for family therapy

Pre-therapy phase:

- Family values
- Cultural values
- Extended family ties
- Kinship circles
- Mate selection
- Parent–child relationships
- Sibling relationships
- Interracial marriages
- Divorce implications
- Remarriage implications
- Impact of migration
- Cultural identity
- Help-seeking patterns

Box 2.23 Therapy process

- Communication principle behaviour – theory
- Communication practice behaviour – practice
- Awareness of family structure theory – engaging the family, cultural interaction, mutual goal setting, selecting a focus system
- Problem-solving phase – directive vs non-directive, social/moral/organic reframing, restructuring social support
- Evaluation and termination

Box 2.24 Additional considerations for therapy

- Man to nature/environment – man with nature or vs nature
- Tune orientation – emphasis on past/present/future
- Relations with people – individual vs social
- Preferred mode of activity – doing vs becoming

In addition to standard family therapy, the therapist should be aware of culturally relevant techniques and skills for specific therapy modules such as marital therapy (see Boxes 2.25 and 2.26). In situations where divorce is occurring, the therapist can still work with the couple and the family to minimize the trauma. In certain cultural settings, single parent or reconstituted family therapies may be indicated.

Box 2.25 Assessing gender roles: some questions

- What does being female mean to you?
- What does your being female mean to your family? Illustrate with examples from partner – parents (father/mother), siblings (male/female), other
- How do their expectations make you feel?
- Ideally what would you like your role to be?
- How does your being female impact on your relationships (with your partner, your parents, your siblings, others)?
- In which way do you think their reactions (partner, parents, siblings, others) to you are to do with your gender?

Box 2.26 Assessing relationship quality

- Who would you approach first to discuss it if something is bothering you?
- How open are you regarding your feelings?
- Are you able to discuss all your problems?
- Do you expect emotional support?
- Do you expect practical support?
- Which do you generally prefer?
- How does that make you feel?
- Are you able to return the feelings?

Non-specific therapies

Of the non-specific therapies, counselling is probably the most commonly used and abused in the UK. Ivey *et al.* (1993) suggest that the following four theories are common in foundational theories of counselling and therapy:

1. A belief in multiple approaches to the helping process
2. An emphasis on multicultural issues

3. The ability to operate as a separate and distinct means of help

4. An emphasis on those underlying processes believed to be important to all approaches to helping.

Empathy, unconditional positive regard and warmth are some of the essential components. Empathy is the process of seeing the world through the eyes of another or hearing as they might hear and feeling and experiencing their internal world. The constructs of empathy include positive attitude and hope for the clients. For multicultural counselling, empathy and positive regard must not be seen as patronizing or controlling. Positive regard focuses on the world view and attitudes towards those whose culture and world view may well differ from us. The empathy rating discussed by Carkhuff (1969) suggests that there are seven levels of empathy, and it is only at a certain level that accurate reflection of feeling, paraphrase or summary catches the essence of what the client says in the clinic. Below this level the counsellor is overtly or subtly destructive, and above this the therapist starts to add interpretation and facilitation of growth and exploration. The pinnacle of counselling is where the therapist is 'with' the client but distinct and apart. Very few therapists achieve this level of empathy.

The questions that therapists may need to address themselves are shown in Box 2.27. These suggest that therapists' personal reflections make an important contribution to the therapeutic relationship. While using empathy, the therapist must clarify some of the underlying issues. These include listening to and observing the client's comments, responding to their constructs, and checking out one's own interventions.

Box 2.27 Therapists' self-examination

- List your ethnic heritage

- Are you monocultural, bicultural or of mixed culture?

- What messages do you receive from each cultural group you have listed?

- How do these messages influence your therapeutic work, especially the approach to clients?

- How well do you recognize your abilities and those of the client?

- How aware are you of discrepancies between your and the client's world view?

Another suggestion put forward by Ivey *et al.* (1993) is that clinicians must try and examine the films and videotapes of interview sessions. They argue that in a successful, smoothly flowing interview, 'movement symmetry' or 'movement complementarity' often occurs between client and counsellor. This is represented by a 'passing' of movement back and forth between the therapeutic dyad. In movement symmetry, counsellor and client assume the same physical posture without being conscious of it, and their eye-to-eye contact is direct. Such a symmetry can be achieved by 'mirroring' the gestures of the client. This mirroring of non-verbal behaviour allows the therapist to be aware and closer to understanding the client.

Basic listening skills in counselling in general and psychotherapy in particular consist of using appropriate open and closed questions; encouraging; paraphrasing; reflection of feeling and summarization. Ivey *et al.* (1993) proposed that influencing skills in the therapeutic encounter include interpretation reframe, directive, information giving, self-disclosure and feedback. For multicultural therapy, a balance must be reached between the individual, family and multicultural issues, and basic listening skills are used to facilitate client understanding of self-in-system. The key themes must be followed in five steps (although it is not essential that these steps occur consecutively):

1. Establishing rapport and structure

2. Gathering data and identifying assets

3. Determining outcomes

4. Generating alternative solutions

5. Generating and transferring learning.

Box 2.28 illustrates Fukuyama's (1990) transcultural universal approach to multicultural counselling. Within such an approach to counselling, the black or cultural identity must be established.

Box 2.28 Fukuyama's (1990) model of transcultural counselling

- Define culture broadly (including gender, ethnicity, race etc.)
- Teach the dangers of stereotyping
- Emphasize the importance of language
- Encourage loyalty and pride in one's own culture
- Inform on acculturation
- Discuss importance of gender roles
- Facilitate identity development
- Build self-esteem and strengths
- Facilitate understanding of one's own world view and its relationship with family and cultural history

In working with families, more than one perspective will be required. Here a sense of integration is essential in developing an understanding of the multiple perspectives on the family, and in addition making sense of the different ways in which the same problem is perceived. The best way to make progress and avoid relapses is to develop and use a network of interventions in order to mix and match approaches within the family setting. Multilevel interventions are required to support and maintain client change. A mixture of psychoanalytic, cognitive, behavioural or intercultural therapies may be required.

Family therapy across cultures has to be directed at the system of conflict, anxiety and defence within the individual and/or the family. For families undergoing processes of acculturation and survival in a mainstream yet possibly or perceptibly hostile society, cultural values must be the focus from which to begin the therapeutic process. Within the assessment processes, the therapist, having identified nuclear versus joint or individualist versus collectivist view on the culture, needs to understand the role of and process of mate selection. Within the family setting, preferred mode of activity, parent–child relationships, parental and child roles and expectations (both individually and socially defined), sibling roles and relationships, divorce and remarriage have to be understood.

Family therapy with ethnic minorities must recognize the impacts of immigration, political discrimination and cultural adjustments. The therapists' role includes not only therapy, but also education, translation, mediation and a model to help families form an open system with available community resources. Communication within the family, between the therapist and the family and between the therapist and the family unit is of prime importance (Figure 2.9).

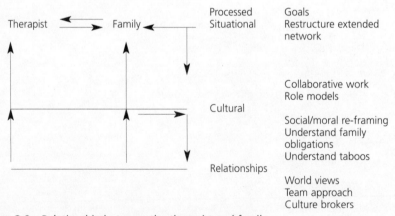

Figure 2.9   Relationship between the therapist and family

The therapist must be prepared to be innovative in order to look at single parent therapy, reconstituted family therapy, divorce work or marital work. A close examination of different ethnic minority groups and the family structures and groupings within them suggests strongly that although the family therapy model based upon white middle-class values may be helpful, it can at times be inappropriate, ineffective and sometimes even harmful. The differences include the extent to which ethnic minority families struggle with or are continuing to struggle with social, economic and political discrimination, unemployment, poor housing, acculturation problems etc. Ethnic minority groups too are heterogeneous, as are members within the same group.

Family therapists must be even more skilled in identifying multifaceted, multilayered processes of acculturation and cultural identity development and formation within each family they come across. Therapists must be sensitive and flexible in their approaches, and Ho (1987) advocates that sessions at home rather than other settings must be the rule rather than the exception. The focus on processes rather than structures within the family is important, and flexibility within such an approach allows the therapist to work with family members.

References

d'Ardenne, P. (1986). Sexual dysfunction in a transcultural setting. *Sexual Marital Therapy* 1, 23–34.

Bhugra, D. and Cordle, C. (1986). Sexual dysfunction in Asian couples. *BMJ* **292**, 111–12.

Bhugra, D. and Cordle, C. (1987). Sexual dysfunction in Asian couples: a case control study. *Sexual Marital Therapy* 3, 69–75.

Bhugra, D. and Bhui, K. (1998). Psychotherapy for ethnic minorities: issues context and practice. *Br. J. Psychotherapy* **14**, 310–26.

Bloom, L. (1991). The dangers of groupism in psychotherapy and counselling. *Freud Museum Offprints*. No. 2. London: Freud Museum.

Carkhuff, R. (1969). *Helping and Human Relations vols 1 & 2*. Troy, M. O.: Holt, Rineheart & Winston.

Carter, R. T. (1995). *The Influence of Race and Racial Identity in Psychotherapy*. NY: John Wiley.

Crowe, M. J. and Ridley, J. (1990). *Therapy with Couples*. Oxford: Blackwell's.

Fukuyama, M. (1990). Taking a universal approach to multicultural counselling. *Counsellor Education and Supervision* **30**, 6–17.

Gupta, P., Bannerjee, G. and Nandi, D. N. (1989): Modified Masters and Johnson technique of sexual inadequacy in males. *2nd J. Psychiat.* **31**, 63–9.

Ho, M. K. (1987). *Family Therapy with Ethnic Minorities*. Palo Alto, C. A.: Sage.

Ivey, A. E., Ivey, M. B. and Simek-Morgan, L. (1993). *Counselling and Psychotherapy*. Boston: Allyn & Bacon.

Kleinman, A. (1980). *Patients and their Healers in the Context of Culture*. Berkeley, CA: Union of California Press.

Lloyd, K. and Bhugra, D. (1993). Cross-cultural aspects of psychotherapy. *Int. Rev. of Psych.* **5**, 291–304.

MacCarthy, B. (1998). Clinical work with ethnic minorities. In: M. F. Walts (ed), *New Developments in Clinical Psychology*. Chichester: John Wiley, pp. 122–39.

Oei, L. and Goh, Y.-W. (1998). Issues in the application of behaviour therapy and constructive behaviour therapy in Asia. In: M. T. P. S. Oei (ed), *Behaviour Therapy and Cognitive Behaviour Therapy in Asia*. Glebe, NSW: Edumedia, 7–14.

Ridley, C. R. (1995). *Overcoming Unintentional Racism in Counselling and Therapy.* Thousand Oaks, CA: Sage.

Suigh, R. S. and Khan, R. (1998). Behaviour therapy in Malaysia. In: M. T. P. S. Oei (ed), *Behaviour Therapy and Cognitive Behaviour Therapy in Asia.* Glebe, NSW: Edumedia, pp. 113–19.

Totman, R. (1982). Philosophical foundations of contribution therapies. In: M. C. Antaki and C. Brewini (eds), *Attributions and Psychological Change.* London: Academic Press.

Tseng, W.S. and McDermott, J. F. (1981). *Culture, Mind and Therapy: an Introduction to Cultural Psychiatry.* NY: Brunner/Mazel.

Turner, S. M. (1982). Introduction. In: M. S. M. Turner and R. J. Jones (eds), *Behaviour modification in Black population: Psychosocial Issues and Empirical Findings.* NY: Plenum.

Walsh, R. N. and Vaughn, F. E. (1980). *Comparative Models of the Person and Psychotherapy.* Palo Alto, CA: Science and Behaviour Books.

Westermeyer, J. (1989). *Psychiatric Care of Migrants: A Clinical Guide.* Washington, DC: APA Press.

Wolberg, L. R. (1997). *The Technique of Psychotherapy.* NY: Grune & Stratton.

Wooding, S. and Oei, T. P. (1998). Cross-socio-cultural diagnosis of mood disorders using DSM IV: its application to aboriginal Australia. In M. T. P. S. Oei (ed): *Behaviour Therapy and Cognitive Behaviour Therapy in Asia.* Glebe, NSW: Edumedia, pp. 17–29.

Yamamoto, J., Silva, J. A., Justice, L. R., Change, C. Y. and Leong, G. (1993). Cross-cultural psychotherapy. In: A. C. Gaw (ed), *Culture, Ethnicity and Mental Illness.* Washington, DC: APA Press, pp. 101–24.

Ethnicity and psychopharmacology

3

Introduction

Although a vast majority of neuroleptics and antidepressants have been developed in the West, drug trials in the initial stages may well be conducted in developing countries and very often little attention is paid to the biological and ethical dimensions of such research. It is only in the last two decades that issues of informed consent and ethnic variations have started to be discussed in the West – especially in the USA. A considerable body of literature is beginning to emerge. The usage of most of these psychiatric drugs is world wide, but substantial differences in their metabolism and in the pharmacological and side effects of these drugs are often ignored while prescribing. It appears that the universalist prescriptive view of the prescribing clinician (which may not always be a psychiatrist) appears to ignore relativist needs of pharmacotherapy. In addition to biological factors directly associated with race and ethnicity, additional cultural factors play a key role in influencing drug compliance and response. The use of alternative health care systems, folk remedies and pluralistic approaches to health care also play a role in the drug response.

Ethnicity

General factors

The definitions of ethnicity, race and culture have already been touched upon in earlier chapters. Ethnicity itself is a product of race, racial characteristics (which have biological factors) and social ascription. At the individual and personal level, individuals can see themselves as belonging to a group with common geographical origins, language and religion and ties, which transcend kinship ties. In addition, traditions, values, religious taboos, folk music, folk memory and folk tales are all shared experiences and can affect an individual's ethnic identity. The wide range of features involved in defining and understanding ethnicity also highlight both the social and biological factors that will influence acceptance of certain kinds of medication and interaction with food and other substances. The use of ethnicity as an epidemiological variable and the role of the clinician as a power in the interaction between patient and clinician have already been touched upon. In this chapter the reader's attention is drawn to personality and metabolic factors in relationship with ethnicity.

Personality factors

Within ethnic groups various social factors such as social and cultural distinctiveness are important. Lin (1996) argues that little is known regarding the potential contribution of cultural and ethnic factors in determining whether a particular drug regime will be of help in treating a particular patient with a specific clinical condition. This neglect of understanding the biological diversity of humankind has led to slow progress in cross-cultural psychiatry regarding factors that influence metabolism. Not taking these factors into account while prescribing has led to a blunderbuss approach in medicating patients from other cultures and minority ethnic groups. The blind acceptance of prescribing guidelines that have been developed for the majority white population whose diet and metabolic factors can be very different to those of patients elsewhere in the world may have no, or only limited, relevance to the latter patients. This Eurocentric and Caucaso-centric approach may have harmed patients in minority or non-European cultures. Individual factors such as height, weight, body mass, body fat and gastric acidity are all related to influences of race and culture, are known to affect the pharmacokinetics of drugs. Culturally determined personality traits (such as interdependence or independence, orthodoxy or adventureness) or subjective responses are all important components of pharmacodynamics and pharmacokinetics which need to be understood along with ethnicity (Lin *et al.*, 1995).

Environmental factors

Additional factors that may influence both pharmacokinetics and pharmacodynamics include the use of caffeine, nicotine, food additives, over-the-counter medications, herbal remedies, environmental pollution etc. (Westermeyer, 1989). Social and family support, personal responses to stress and coping strategies will also influence the prognosis and outcome of treatment of the mentally ill. People with higher levels of stress and lower levels of social support have been noted to have poor social and clinical outcomes, and these levels have been postulated to influence therapeutic dosages and therapeutic levels of different medications. The role of the family in compliance and adherence, either directly or through expressed emotion, needs to be investigated further. Smith and Mendoza (1996) suggest that environmental factors may influence the underlying genetic factors that in turn cause ethnic differences in the genetic structure of drug-metabolizing enzymes, which would explain the differences in pharmocological responses linked with ethnic factors.

Traditional remedies

Many ethnic groups will use 'traditional' or non-Western remedies. Some of these schools of medicine are well established, such as Ayurveda, Unani or homeopathy, whereas other patients may resort to remedies from health food shops or herbalists. Many of these remedies contain higher doses of psychoactive substances, which can lead to significant interactions with prescribed drugs. Both Ayurvedic and Unani medications may well contain high levels of lead, mercury, antimony, gold, silver, tin, copper or zinc. In addition, health practitioners from these schools may well recommend food taboos and dietary restrictions, which will influence the absorption of food and medication. Several ethnic groups, especially from the Indian subcontinent, will use pluralistic approaches, and such information may not be readily made available to the clinician. The clinician must ask for information in these areas in a sensitive and careful manner.

Pharmacodynamics

Pharmacodynamics is the study of the effects a drug has on an organism. It refers to the neurotransmitter, neurophysiological, behavioural, psychological and social effects of psychotropic drugs and their mechanisms of action. A common example, highlighted by Westermeyer (1989), is the flushing response to alcohol seen among Chinese individuals. Such a response has a variable distribution across races due to the differences in enzymes acting on alcohol metabolism. Although the mechanics of alcohol flushing have been well described, the relationships between differences in blood levels, therapeutic responses and dosages are not well understood. Westermeyer (1989) suggests that these differences may be due to (but not limited to) the following factors:

1. Pharmacokinetic factors, such as enzymatic differences

2. Pharmacodynamic factors, such as variable neurotransmitter systems

3. Social and psychological differences, such as variations in tolerance to symptoms across cultures

4. Differences in clinical practice, such as availability of laboratory facilities

5. Sampling problems

6. Methodological problems.

A clear example of ethnic factors influencing pharmacodynamics is demonstrated by the greater sensitivity to mydriatics in Caucasians rather than Asians or in African-Americans (Lin *et al.*, 1984).

Pharmacogenetic traits significantly affect the pharmacokinetics of a number of psychotropics, and are likely to be clinically important.

Pharmocokinetics

Pharmacokinetics is the study of how a biological organism affects the fate and distribution of a drug. This is determined by four processes: absorption, distribution, metabolism and excretion. The process of metabolism exhibits cross-ethnic as well as individual differences. Differences in height, weight, gastric acidity, body mass and body fat all play an important role in influencing the pharmacokinetics of drugs, and these are in turn influenced by race and ethnicity. The influences of social and environmental factors on various ethnic factors are shown in Figure 3.1.

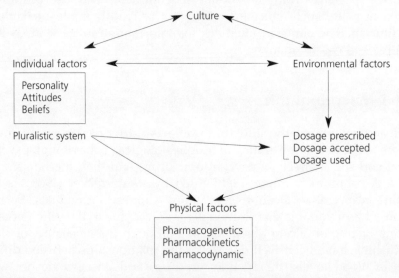

Figure 3.1   Inter-relationship of individual and cultural factors.

Mechanisms affecting pharmacological response

Lin *et al.* (1995) have suggested that drugs, as well as other foreign substances (xenobiotics), are metabolized by a number of enzymes whose activities may vary substantially across individuals and ethnic groups both for genetic and environmental reasons (see Box 3.1). Even though individual and inter-ethnic differences are substantial, the mechanisms that are responsible for such variations have been less well understood (Lin *et al.*, 1993). In addition to classical examples of drug responses across ethnic groups, the genetic control of a large number of drug metabolizing enzymes has been established. For example, the cytochrome P-450 enzyme system has been linked with oxidation of several chemotherapeutic agents. More than 20 P-450 isoenzymes exist, and each is encoded by a specific gene. Both the phenotypes and genotypes of this enzyme system show clear individual and cross-ethnic variations, which have been linked with differential adaptation to divergent environmental exposure – especially diet. Clear diversity is seen, with some P-450 isoenzymes leading to poor or good metabolism. Lin *et al.* (1993) reported that the ethnic variations of these enzymes range from 1 per cent in East Asians to 8.1 per cent in American blacks. Other enzymes also show a similar range of variation. Individual P-450 isoenzymes involved in the metabolism of psychiatric drugs include CYP1A2, CYP2C, CYP2D6 and CYP3A4. Of these, CYP2D6 is particularly involved in the metabolism of haloperidol, perphenazine, risperidone and thioridazine. Individuals possessing a mutation at the CYP2D6 isoenzyme are referred to as poor metabolizers, whereas individuals possessing a normally functioning enzyme are referred to as extensive metabolizers. Poor metabolizers may accumulate potentially toxic blood concentrations following the administration of standard dosages dependent on the CYP2D6 isoenzyme. Frackiewicz *et al.* (1997) suggested that research confirms, in spite of methodological problems, fairly consistent differences in response to antipsychotic medication, with certain ethnically defined populations requiring lower dosages of antipsychotics. Similarly, beta-blockers have been shown to be relatively ineffective in treating hypertension in African-Americans, but are said to be more effective in Asians, with responses in Caucasians falling somewhere in the middle. In the same way, clozapine-induced agranulocytosis has been most commonly observed in Ashkenazi Jews, especially in those with a special cluster of HLA antigen (Lieberman *et al.*, 1990).

Box 3.1 Planning pharmacotherapy

• Prior to prescribing	Check diet
	Check dietary taboos
	Check religious taboos
	Check alcohol, caffeine, nicotine intake
• While prescribing	Start at lowest dose
	Use low threshold for identifying side effects
	Adjust dosages slowly
	Make information freely available to patients and carers
• After prescribing	Monitor side effects
	Check compliance
	Check complementary medications

Ethnic differences

Most of the data available on ethnicity and psychopharmacology have been reported from the USA, and of all the psychotropics, neuroleptics and antidepressants have been studied at length.

NEUROLEPTICS

Cross-racial differences in the doses of neuroleptics that produce side effects have been studied extensively in Asian-Americans (those of Far-Eastern Asian ancestry or descent, including but not limited to Chinese, Japanese, Korean, Vietnamese, Thais and Filipinos) and non-Hispanic Caucasian populations in the USA. Postulated mechanisms for these ethnic/racial differences include pharmacokinetic and pharmacodynamic variations, and non-pharmacological explanations such as cultural and societal variations in the way psychiatry is practised (Frackiewicz et al., 1997).

ENZYMES

As noted above, cytochrome P-450 isoenzymes play a key role in the variability of drug response because these enzymes are involved in the oxidative metabolism of a wide range of xenobiotics. Those individuals who possess a normally functioning enzyme are referred to as extensive metabolizers, compared with those who have experienced mutation at the CYP2D6 locus by virtue of lacking a functional form of the CYP2D6 isoenzyme and are poor metabolizers. Poor metabolizers are thus likely to accumulate potentially toxic serum concentration levels even if they are given standard doses of substrates dependent on the CYP2D6 isoenzyme, thereby producing a much higher level of side effects. It has been suggested that 6–10 per cent of Caucasians in Europe and North America have the mutation at the CYP2D6 isoenzyme level, causing poor metabolism of drugs degraded by this enzyme, whereas the rate is less than 1 per cent in Japan, China and other parts of Far East Asia. The frequency of poor metabolizers in African populations varies considerably, from 0.7–5 per cent for Ghanaians, 3–8 per cent for Nigerians and as high as 18 per cent for Sam Bushmen. Other studies show rates of 7.7 per cent among Caucasians and 1.9 per cent for African-Americans, and for Hispanics the figure appears to be 4.5 per cent (see Frackiewicz et al., 1997). These authors suggest that genetic polymorphism is complex and alterations at the DNA level may result in CYP2D6 activity, which is absent (poor metabolizers), increased (ultra-rapid metabolism) or decreased (slow metabolizers) compared with the homozygous form of the enzyme.

DIETARY, ENVIRONMENTAL AND OTHER FACTORS

Dosage studies and ethnic differences in antipsychotic adverse effects suggest that there are clear inter-ethnic and intra-ethnic differences that clinicians must be aware of (see Figure 3.1). As mentioned earlier, concomitant smoking, alcohol and exposure to occupational or environmental toxins may also influence drug elimination rates.

Smoking is known to cause enzyme induction in humans, leading to increased clearance and decreased concentration of a number of drugs. It has been suggested that smokers who smoke more than one packet of cigarettes a day have significantly lower concentrations of haloperidol than non-smokers. The clearance of haloperidol has been shown to be greater in smokers. Similarly, effects on chlorpromazine and fluphenazine levels have been noted in response to smoking. The prevalence studies of smoking in normal populations and specific ethnic groups have shown varying rates of smoking and caffeine intake. Frackiewicz *et al.* (1997) suggested that the lower incidence of smoking in some ethnic groups like African-Americans and Mexican-Americans may result in higher plasma antipsychotic drug concentrations, leading to increased sensitivity to drug effects. Similarly, the use of caffeine in coffee, tea and cola drinks can interfere with drug metabolism. The two key inter-ethnic metabolic differences that have been highlighted in response to caffeine are:

1. The genetic acetylator status, which affects the fate of paraxanthine (the main metabolite of caffeine), although this does not affect the rate of elimination of caffeine itself

2. The urinary metabolism of paraxanthine, although it is not clear whether this is affected at metabolic or renal transport levels.

In a study of the five metabolites of caffeine (Kalow, 1986a), there were statistically significant differences in at least two metabolites between Oriental and Caucasian subjects living in Canada. Kalow (1986a) reported that ethnic differences of the metabolite profile seemed to show in a difference in appearance rates of 17 per cent, indicating either an increased rate of formation in Caucasians or an increased rate of urinary elimination in Orientals. Kalow (1986b) suggests that genetic variations in response to diverse tasting abilites for phenylthiocarbamide vary. For example, most European populations have 25 per cent non-tasters, Hindu populations about 33 per cent and Brazilian Indians only 1 per cent. The epidemiological association between tasting ability and thyroid disease is well established. Genetic variations on insensitivity to other tastes and smells have been well established.

Kalow (1986a) argues that a study of caffeine metabolites reveals two kinds of inter-ethnic variations pertaining to the well known acetylation polymorphism affecting the secondary metabolism of the parent drug and differences in paraxanthine excretion, which may be related to ethnic differences in renal function. The levels of caffeine may well interact with levels of other drugs and increase or decrease levels of metabolites, thereby causing side effects to be major problems. Furthermore, caffeine and smoking may each contribute to the additive factors.

Body weight, age and diet are also factors that influence the metabolism of various drugs. Body weight and body fat influence serum plasma concentrations of different drugs, and people with a low body weight may require lower dosage levels to achieve the same plasma concentrations Dosage adjustments should not be made on the basis of the body surface area. In obese individuals, levels of highly lipophilic drugs like haloperidol are increased, necessitating higher doses. The types of obesity in different ethnic groups may therefore influence absorption as well as the levels of drugs.

Age is one of the key and well-established factors that has been shown to influence metabolism and absorption, and hence drug dosages. Some of these changes are attributable to body composition, protein binding and renal clearance. These factors tend to be influenced by an ageing liver and changes in diet and lifestyle.

Diet affects the pharmacokinetics of drugs. Some foods (especially vegetables like cabbage, broccoli and Brussels sprouts) are potent inducers of chemical oxidation, and increase the expression of CYP1A2. Diets high in these substances decrease the systematic availability of some drugs such as the antipsychotics haloperidol and clozapine. Polycyclic aromatic hydrocarbons formed during charcoal broiling also contribute to enhanced drug oxidation rates. Grapefruit juice (even in quantities as small as 200ml) can inhibit the CYP1A2 and causes clinically meaningful increases in the serum concentration of certain medications. The amount of protein and carbohydrate consumed in the diet may affect P-450 enzymes and alter the rates of metabolism of drugs that are substrates of P-450 isoenzymes. High protein and low carbohydrate diets can decrease the half-life of certain analgesics by increasing their elimination. Because the availability of types of food may vary, different levels of acculturation may lead to different patterns of diet and metabolism. Some components in Chinese dishes, and Chinese herbal medicines such as ginseng, can induce cytochrome P-450 enzymes, and thus have the potential for significant long interactions. Clinicians must therefore be aware of these specific issues when dealing with specific ethnic groups.

An additional point raised by Frackiewicz *et al.* (1997) is the role of drugs in crossing blood–brain barriers, where they interact with central nervous system receptors. As only the unbound fraction is able to cross the blood–brain barrier, even minute variations in the concentration of drug-binding proteins could lead to massive differences in response and side effects. The level of binding to α2-acid glycoprotein is significantly reduced in the Chinese subjects, and as the glycoprotein binds to several neuroleptics such as haloperidol, chlorpromazine, fluphenazine and thioridazine, the differences in dosage required to reach the same levels in the Chinese become very important. Cross-racial differences in the doses of neuroleptics have been studied extensively in Asian-Americans. Binder and Levy (1981) reported that 95 per cent of Asians in their sample had developed extrapyramidal side effects within 2 weeks of commencing treatment, compared with 60 per cent of blacks and 67 per cent of whites on equivalent dosages. Even though the numbers in this study are relatively small, these remain significant differences. Jann et al. (1989) also reported that the Chinese had higher levels of extra pyramidal side effects when commenced on haloperidol. Chang et al. (1991) found that reduced haloperidol ratios were generally lower among Chinese when compared with non-Chinese subjects, suggesting that different metabolic factors may well be at play.

Using healthy volunteers, Midha et al. (1989) were able to demonstrate that lower haloperidol levels were seen among more black individuals than white individuals. These authors gave single doses (5mg) of haloperidol to 26 black and 10 white healthy men, of whom 22 and 6 respectively completed the study. Plasma haloperidol samples were analysed for haloperidol and reduced haloperidol over a 36-hour period, and reduced haloperidol was detectable in only five blacks and one white. They also found that there was a widespread inter-subject variation in the area under the plasma concentration versus time curve. They conclude that these wide variations could result from a number of reasons. Lin and Poland (1984), on the other hand, found that Asian-Americans had significantly higher serum levels on haloperidol, and also had a more pronounced prolactive response when compared with the white group. The lower ratios of reduced haloperidol and haloperidol levels in Asian-Americans have been postulated to be due to slower rates of reduction and metabolism. Lin et al. (1988) were able to demonstrate higher serum haloperidol levels in healthy Americans of Far-Eastern Asian descent when compared with white volunteers, and a later study confirmed this, suggesting that Asian-Americans with schizophrenia were more likely to respond to low doses of haloperidol. These findings have not yet been confirmed in other ethnic groups, but if they are, clinicians will have to alter their clinical practice and prescribing habits. Further clinical and research evidence is required to elucidate whether drug interactions are associated with specific compounds or neurotransmitters as well as interactions with food, diet and other environmental factors.

PHARMACODYNAMIC HYPOTHESES

It is theoretically possible that different ethnic or racial groups may well have altered affinity with different neuroceptors, thereby requiring different levels of drugs. Ethnic differences in the dopamine D2 receptors have recently been discovered, although these have not been shown to be associated with schizophrenia or even antipsychotic drug response. Further efforts are therefore required to confirm relativist biological factors in different ethnic groups.

PRESCRIBING FACTORS

Although, as Frackiewicz *et al.* (1997) argue, dose–response relationships for antipsychotics have not been demonstrated and lower dosages of antipsychotics are as effective in treatment as higher doses, low dosages of haloperidol (2mg per day) have been shown to result in high concentration of D2 receptor occupancy in the region of 53–74 per cent (Kapur *et al.*, 1996). These authors recommend that clinicians should be encouraged to commence treatment on small doses. In some countries, e.g. Japan, low dosages are recommended, as well as a combination of antipsychotics. Ethnic differences in prescribed doses are also likely to be influenced by social and economic factors. In India, for example, a mixture of antipsychotic drugs will be used in clinical practice. It is also likely that, once clinicians believe that a particular group should receive less medication, they will change their prescribing habits. However, some ethnic groups (e.g. African-Caribbeans in the UK) may be more likely to be diagnosed as having high rates of schizophrenia and are therefore likely to be treated with significantly higher dosages of antipsychotic agents. Frackiewicz *et al.* (1997) caution that the prescribing habits of clinicians may well be more important than actual differences in response. Specific factors related to treatment adherence and compliance are likely to play an important role as well.

DOSAGES OF ANTIPSYCHOTICS

As mentioned earlier, in certain conditions and certain countries the mean daily doses of antipsychotics are lower than recommended for the Western patients. Chiu *et al.* (1992) reported that the mean daily dose of antipsychotics was two to three times lower for Chinese patients than that prescribed by the American psychiatrists to Caucasian patients, even after differences in body weight had been taken into account. Lin *et al.* (1995) cite that, when Asian and Caucasian patients with psychosis had been matched on age, diagnosis, duration of illness and past antipsychotic exposure, Asian patients required significantly lower dosages of antipsychotic medication than did Caucasians in order to control the symptoms.

When Asian patients with the diagnosis of schizophrenia and normal volunteers were given comparable doses of medication, the former showed approximately 50 per cent greater metabolic rates then their Caucasian counterparts (Lin *et al.*, 1995). The mechanisms said to be responsible for such ethnic differences are related to a number of genetic and metabolic factors. Asian patients (in this case largely Korean, Japanese, Chinese and Taiwanese) with schizophrenia respond optimally to significantly lower plasma haloperidol concentrations as compared with their Caucasian counterparts. The differences between black and white Americans are not as clear cut, and neither are the data for Hispanic Americans.

Tardive dyskinesia is a side effect of the long-term use of neuroleptics, and its prevalence in Western samples has varied from 0.5 to 65 per cent, with an average prevalence of 20 per cent. Advanced age and female gender have been identified as two key factors that make risk of tardive dyskinesia more likely. Pi *et al.* (1993) illustrated that rates of tardive dyskinesia varied from 8.4 per cent in China to 20.6 per cent in Japan. In a multi-national study of tardive dyskinesia in Asians, Pi *et al.* (1990) reported an overall prevalence of 17 per cent; however, the Chinese in China had the lowest rate at 8.2 per cent, whereas rates among Koreans and Chinese were broadly similar in Hong Kong and Yanji. Multiple regression analysis identified key risk factors as being over the age of 50 years, the current neuroleptic dose and the geographical region (for those outside Beijing the risk was lower than for those in Beijing). Although several methodological problems remain, these findings suggest that there are geographical and ethnic variations of which the clinicians must be aware.

As tardive dyskinesia does not have a safe or effective treatment, prevention is the major aim regardless of a patient's culture. The prescription of neuroleptics should be clinically indicated, and the lowest possible dosages should be adhered to.

Binder and Levy (1981) showed that a greater percentage of Asian patients who were on haloperidol developed extra pyramidal symptoms when compared with blacks or whites. Similar findings have also been reported by other authors, but studies assessing ethnic/racial differences in the incidence of tardive dyskinesia are not conclusive.

Ethnic differences have been reported regarding other adverse effects as well. For example, Ashkenazi Jews on clozapine are more likely to develop agranulocytosis compared with others.

ANTIDEPRESSANTS

The results of studies on ethnic differences in the pharmocokinetics of tricyclic antidepressants have been less conclusive. Lin *et al.* (1995) illustrated this by citing six studies, of which three showed that in comparisons between Asians and whites, the former group metabolize tricyclic antidepressants more slowly than the latter. Other studies showed similar but insignificant differences. The results of differences among ethnic groups are less conclusive. Allen *et al.* (1977), Lewis *et al.* (1980) and Rudorfer *et al.* (1984) have reported that Caucasians appear to have lower plasma levels of tricyclic antidepressants and attain plasma peak levels later when compared with Asians (this comparison included those from the Indian subcontinent as well). These differences have been attributed by Kalow (1982) to the greater incidence of slow hydroxylation among Asians. Gaviria *et al.* (1986) reported that among healthy non-depressed volunteers, purported hypersensitivity to drugs among Hispanics was related to receptor hypersensitivity – this group appeared to respond to lower doses and had more side effects on tricyclic antidepressants.

Studies from Asia itself have demonstrated that severely depressed Asian patients responded to lower combined concentrations of imipramine and desipramine when compared with dosages used for white groups. African-Americans have been reported to have higher than normal levels of neurological side effects due to antidepressants with standard doses. The mechanisms of these actions are far from clear. The dosages of antidepressants should be carefully tailored to individual needs and responses, all the while monitoring side effects. For tricyclic antidepressants, intra-group variations in pharmacokinetics are probably more important than inter-group variations.

The existing data on newer antidepressants and atypical neuroloeptics are scanty, and the dosage of newer antidepressants and assessment of side effects across different ethnic groups deserve to be studied further. It is possible that newer antidepressants such as moclobemide will have higher levels of variation compared with other antidepressants especially because, for monoamine oxidase inhibitors, variations across different ethnic groups are likely to be even more marked.

LITHIUM

Racial differences in red blood cell sodium and lithium levels have been well documented (Westermeyer, 1989). Various pharmacokinetic differences may exist, but the precise nature and its impact on clinical issues is not well described. Among Japanese patients lithium has been proved effective at lower dosages, but among Taiwanese patients higher doses are required to maintain clinical efficacy in comparison with Japanese, although these are lower than in American patients (Chang et al., 1985). Taiwanese patients are maintained at lithium levels of 0.5–0.79mEq/l, whereas Chinese patients are said to respond to levels of around 0.71–0.73mEq/l, even though no pharmacokinetic differences have been reported among Chinese-Americans.

Environmental factors such as the weather, dehydration and diet are more likely to influence lithium levels and produce toxic levels in comparison with other drugs. Lin et al. (1995) reported that higher RBC/plasma lithium ratio in African-Americans and African blacks may lead to higher levels of toxicity, thereby suggesting that their therapeutic serum or plasma lithium concentrations might need to be reduced when compared with patients from other ethnic groups.

BENZODIAZEPINES

The pharmacokinetic differences between ethnic groups regarding response to benzodiazepines are noted to be significant. The rates of metabolism of benzodiazepines (especially diazepam and alprazolam) have been noted to be slower among Asians when compared with white Americans. Studies among Asians were carried out in different geographical locations, suggesting that genetic factors appeared to be more important than environmental factors in controlling benzodiazepine metabolism (Lin *et al.*, 1995). On investigating the effects of adinazolam, African-Americans had notably increased clearance and significantly higher concentrations of its metabolites and greater drug effects on psychomotor performance. These differences have been attributed to hepatic oxidation and renal excretions, which may well explain the greater drug effect on African-Americans despite their higher metabolic capacity for adinazolam.

Other physical treatments and prescribed or non-prescribed drugs such as analgesics may still be used in conjunction with psychotropic drugs, thereby increasing the likelihood of drug interaction. Often individuals from different cultures will use pluralistic approaches to help-seeking, and the clinician must be aware of these.

Non-biological factors

Figure 3.1 illustrates the interaction of the individual, cultural and environmental factors that may be important in the metabolism of drugs, and some of these factors have already been mentioned. However, cultures differ in the way they train and allow their members to be on guard against certain types of mental state and behaviours. Help-seeking follows a clear recognition of symptoms, which are then identified as odd and out of context for the cultural setting so that a cultural meaning can be given and appropriate health care sought. Pluralistic approaches, geographical and economic access to help providers and complementary therapies are all-important factors in determining the response to drugs.

Stress

Stress and social support both play an important role in compliance and the response to drugs. Alterations in stress levels and altered social support will determine compliance, the prognosis and the outcome. Any continuing stress may suggest that individuals or their carers may well be using other stress-reducing mechanisms – for example, refugees may be dealing with ongoing stress and lack of social support by using potions that they may be familiar with from their country of origin.

The role of gender in pharmacological response has only recently been studied (Dawkins, 1996). Gender determines expectations, social support and compliance. Dawkins (1996) argues that the interaction between gender and ethnicity, patient information, risk factors and accurate diagnosis is all-important in successful clinical psychopharmacology.

Lee (1993) observed that in Hong Kong, Chinese physicians have a paternalistic relationship with their patients and are expected to treat patients with kindness. In return, patients are expected to be deferential and compliant and not to question the indications for lithium treatment or for regular blood tests. Lee (1993) reported that, of 70 patients who were on lithium and asked about side effects, only nine (20 per cent) of those who reported side effects acknowledged polydipsia and polyuria to be troublesome. These side effects were generally seen as positive in that water excretion and consumption were important in ridding the body of toxins and aiding digestion. In contrast with Western patients, Chinese bipolar patients rarely mourned the loss of expansive mood, creativity or extroversion associated with bipolar moods. This acceptance was linked with the restraint and introversion expected of the Chinese culture.

For women, factors such as body weight, height and hormonal changes are likely to affect pharmocokinetics and pharmacodynamics. The role of gender in help-seeking has been studied, and it suggests that women are more likely to be responsible for help-seeking for others but often neglect themselves, especially in some patriarchal cultures. The role of alcohol, smoking, caffeine intake and other factors will also differ according to gender. Gender combined with age and ethnicity is likely to play a very important role in compliance and drug response.

The role of culture in forming the personality and the interaction between personality traits and drug response is very important. Murphy (1969) suggested that, when compared to those imbued with a culture giving a strong emphasis to independence, struggle and action, patients with cultural backgrounds emphasizing interdependence and social adaptation would require less medication in general. This was further confirmed by Murphy (1972) when he reported that ethnic Chinese patients with schizophrenia were less responsive to neuroleptics when compared to their native Indonesian counterparts (Malays are generally regarded as less aggressive and action-oriented than Chinese), and two anxiolytics were more effective clinically but led to more side effects in French-Canadians than in Anglo-Canadians.

Several other authors have confirmed this. Those patients who respond in an orthodox manner (i.e. with sedation) to neuroleptics are likely to be passive and intellectually oriented, whereas patients with paradoxical reactions are likely to be action-oriented and athletically inclined. The responses in the latter group are often characterized by paradoxical increases in agitation, tension and anxiety, leading to increasingly higher doses (see Lin *et al.*, 1995, for a detailed discussion).

Cultural patterns of pluralism

Cross-national differences exist in terms of the type and dosage of medication for similar conditions. These differences are often related to availability and patient expectations as well as to prescribers' beliefs, especially regarding the clinical and untoward effects of the medications. Cultural stereotypes can also influence prescribing patterns – for example, Asian women may be seen as passive and be more likely to be prescribed benzodiazepines although not diagnosed with common mental disorders.

Many cultures use pluralistic approaches, and will happily combine herbs, Ayurvedic or homeopathic medicines with Western medicines. Many of these 'traditional' medicines have pharmacological actions, and are capable of significant drug interactions with prescribed psychiatric drugs. Several of these drugs are rich in lead or other metals.

Placebo response

The placebo phenomenon accounts for 30–70 per cent of the therapeutic response obtained with any treatment method, and although well described it has not been studied extensively – especially across cultures. Diagnosis, colour and size of tablets and method of drug administration all influence the placebo response (see Smith *et al.*, 1993). As the placebo response is mediated not only through a symbolic interaction but also through faith in the therapy, it is likely to be influenced by cultural factors. There is only a limited amount of information available on placebo responses across different cultures. Escobar and Tuason (1980) studied the effects of trazadone and a placebo in 40 Colombian and 32 American depressed patients, and found that Colombian patients improved more on both trazadone and on placebo. Smith *et al.* (1993) suggested that, in spite of a paucity of studies, it appears that non-Caucasians may be somewhat more responsive to placebo treatment. Buckalew and Coffield (1982) reported that white capsules were seen as analgesics by Caucasian subjects but as stimulants by African-Americans, and black capsules were seen in exactly the reverse way. Thus the ethnic and culture-specific nature of these drug effects must be investigated further.

In addition, social support systems, social networks and the quality of support all play an important role in the interaction.

Compliance

Compliance with medication depends upon a number of factors, such as dosage, side effects, past experiences with medication, models of illness and beliefs in health care. Many psychiatric patients will require long-term medication, and their expectations of treatment will vary. Even though treatment packages have been developed to improve compliance, their success in treating patients from other cultures has not been entirely proven. Divergence in the beliefs of patients and clinicians, as well as difficulties in communications, will influence compliance. Appropriate educational packages in appropriate languages will enhance compliance.

Conclusions

This brief overview highlights some of the key issues the clinicians must be aware of, and Box 3.2 summarizes the implementation of the treatment plan. Future research will enable clinicians to be more focused in their approaches when dealing with members of other cultures.

Box 3.2 Implementing the treatment plan

- Convey the diagnosis to the patient and carers
- Convey the recommended intervention
- Discuss the above in easily understandable terms
- Ensure that the patient and carers have understood the diagnosis, treatment and prognosis, with or without treatment
- Discuss the advantages and disadvantages of treatment
- Clarify the expectations of the patient and carers
- Be prepared for follow-up discussion

References

Allen, J., Rack, P. and Vaddadi, K. (1977). Differences in the effects of chloripranine on English and Asian volunteers. *Postgrad. Med. J.*, **53**, 79–86.

Binder, E. and Levy, R. (1981). Extrapyramidal reactions in Asians. *Am. J. Psychiatry*, **138**, 1243–4.

Buckalew, L. and Coffield, K. (1982). Drug expectations associated with perceptual characteristics. *Percept. Motor Skills*, **55**, 915–18.

Chang, S. S., Paney, G., Yan, Y. *et al.* (1985). Lithium pharmacokinetics. Paper presented at APA meeting, Dallas. In K. M. Lin, R. Poland and G. Nakasaki (eds) (1993). *Psychopharmacology and Psychobiology of Ethnicity*. APA Press.

Chang, S., Jann, M., Hsu, H.-G. *et al.* (1991). Ethnic comparison of haloperidol and reduced haloperidol ratios in Chinese patients. *Biol. Psych.*, **22**, 1406–8.

Chiu, H., Sham, P., Lau, J. *et al.* (1992). Prevalence of tardive dyskinesia, tardive dystonia and respiratory dyskinesia in Chinese psychiatric patients in Hong Kong. *Am. J. Psychiatry*, **149**, 1081–5.

Dawkins, L. (1996). The interaction of ethnicity, sociocultural factors and gender in clinical psychopharmacology. *Psychopharmacol. Bull.*, **32**, 283–9.

Escobar, J. and Tuason, V. (1980). Antidepressant agents: a cross-cultural study. *Psychopharmacol. Bull.*, **16**, 49–52.

Frackiewicz, E., Stannek, J., Herrara, J. *et al.* (1997). Ethnicity and antipsychotic response. *Ann. Psychopharmacol.*, **31**, 1360–9.

Gaviria, M., Gill, A. and Javaid, J. (1986). Nortriptyline kinetics in Hispanic and Anglo subjects. *J. Clin. Psychpharmacol.*, **6**, 227–31.

Jann, M., Chang, W., Davis, C. *et al*. (1989). Haloperidol and reduced haloperidol plasma levels in four different ethnic populations. *Prog. Neuropsychopharmacol. Biol. Psych.*, **16**, 193–202.

Kalow, W. (1982). Ethnic differences in drug metabolism. *Clin. Pharmacokinet.*, **71**, 373–400.

Kalow, W. (1986a). Caffeine and other drugs. In: W. Kalow, H. Goedde and D. Agarwal (eds), *Progress in Clinical and Biological* Research, Alan R Liss Inc. 331–41.

Kalow, W. (1986b). Outlook of a pharmacologist. In: W. Kalow, H. Goedde and D. Agarwal (eds), *Progress in Clinical and Biological Research*, Alan R Liss Inc., pp. 3–7.

Kapur, S., Remington, G., Jones, C. *et al*. (1996). High concentrations of dopamine D2 receptor occupancy with low dose haloperidol treatment: a PET study. *Am. J. Psychiatry*, **153**, 948–50.

Lee, S. (1993). Side effects of chronic lithium therapy in Hong Kong Chinese: an ethnopsychiatric perspective. *Cult. Med. Psychiatry*, **17**, 301–20.

Lewis, P., Rack, P., Vaddadi, K. *et al*. (1980). Ethnic differences in drug response. *Postgrad. Med. J.*, **56**, 46–9.

Lieberman, J., Yunis, J., Egla, E. *et al*. (1990). HLA-338, DR4, DRW3 and clozapine-induced agranulocytosis in Jewish patients with schizophrenia. *Arch. Gen. Psych.*, **47**, 945–8.

Lin, K.-M. (1996). Psychopharmacology in cross-cultural psychiatry. *Mt Sinai J. Med.*, **63**, 283–4.

Lin, K.-M. and Poland, R. (1984). Variations in neuroleptic response. Paper presented at meeting of society for the Study of Culture and Psychiatry, Santa Fe.

Lin, K.-M., Lau, J., Smith, R. and Poland, R. (1988). Comparison of alprazolam plasma levels and behavioural effects in normal Asian and Caucasian male volunteers. *Psychopharmacology*, **96**, 365–9.

Lin, K.-M., Poland, R. and Nakasaki, G. (eds) (1993). *Psychopharmacology and Psychobiology of Ethnicity*. APA Press.

Lin, K.-M., Poland, R. and Anderson, D. (1995). Psychopharmacology, ethnicity and culture. *Transcult. Psych. Res. Rev.*, **32**, 3–40.

Midha, K., Chakraborty, B. S., Ganes, D. A. *et al*. (1989). Intersubject variation in the pharmacokinetics of haloperidol and reduced haloperidol. *J. Clin. Psychopharmacol.*, **9**, 98–104.

Murphy, H. B. M. (1969). Ethnic variations in drug response. *Transcult. Psych. Res. Rev.*, **6**, 6–25.

Murphy, H. B. M. (1972). Psychopharmacologie et variations. *Ethnoculturelle Confrontation Psychiatrique*, **90**, 163–85.

Pi, E. H., Gray, G., Lee, S. *et al*. (1990). Tardive dyskinesia in Asians. A multinational study paper presented at the APA meeting, New York.

Pi, E. H., Guttirez, M. and Gray, G. (1993). Tardive dyskinesia: cross-cultural perspectives. In: K.-M. Lin, R. Poland and G. Nakasaki, eds. *Psychopharmacology and Psychobiology of Ethnicity*, APA Press, 153–68.

Rudorfer, E., Lam, E., Chang, W. *et al*. (1984). Desipranine pharmacokinetics in Chinese and Caucasian volunteers. *Br. J. Clin. Pharmacol.*, **17**, 433–40.

Smith, M. and Mendoza, R. (1996). Ethnicity pharmacokinetics. *Mt Sinai J. Med.*, **63**, 285–90.

Smith, M., Lin, K.-M. and Mendoza, R. (1993). 'Non-biological' issues affecting psychopharmacotherapy: cultural considerations. In: K.-M. Lin, R. Poland and G. Nakasaki, eds. *Psychopharmacology and Psychobiology of Ethnicity*. APA Press, 37–58.

Westermeyer, J. (1989). *Psychiatric Care of Migrants: A Clinical Guide*. APA Press.

The following references in Chapter 1 are also relevant to the issues dealt with in this chapter:

Bhugra *et al.* (1997)
Bhugra *et al.* (1999)
Buffenstein (1997)
Castillo (1997)
Hendin (1969)
Ho (1987)
Ivey *et al.* (1993)
Jablensky *et al.* (1992)
Jones and Gray (1986)
Shrout *et al.* (1992)
Tseng (1975)
Tseng (1997)
Tseng and Streltzer (1997)
Ucko (1994)
WHO (1974)

Transcultural psychiatry: generational problems

4

Introduction

The socio-demographic profile of ethnic minority groups in the UK is changing. The younger and in some instances British-born minority ethnic population appears to suffer from higher rates of some psychiatric disorders, and lower rates of others. The exact patterns vary according to the ethnicity, generation, specific traumatic migration histories and adverse life events associated with ethnic minority status.

Migration has been an age-old process of geographical movement from one part of the world to another for social, political, military or economic reasons. With such movements, individuals take their cultural beliefs, values and lifestyles with them. Ethnic identity is often seen as a fixed category to which people assign themselves, rather than a process by which individuals seek a group identity. This identity is then used to contest their needs and to sustain their sense of belonging in the face of adversity. Before migration, individuals may have had an opportunity to think about their ethnic identity; however, it is likely that they thought more about their identity as men or women, or as young people, adults or adolescents with tension between the way people treat them and they way they feel. Migration tends to amplify conflicts of identity by bringing to the fore questions about cultural differences, a sense of belonging or alienation, self worth and social group membership. Social exclusion and oppression can also unite groups that would otherwise consider themselves distinct. Following migration, minority groups have to deal with poorer economic circumstances and housing conditions, ill health, the inability to access services with which they are unfamiliar, occasional disparagement from the dominant community, and stereotypical representations of themselves. These stereotypes include those of racial 'inferiority', 'strange' foods and dress, as well as 'odd' customs that the host population does not understand, value or welcome. Where these host values and behaviours conflict with 'perceived immigrant' values and behaviours, there is potential for conflict if either the host or the perceived immigrant feel compelled to accept values that they find distasteful. Thus, 'arranged marriage' is often talked about as an evil subjugation of one person to be married to another in a manner that Western standards of individual autonomy and self-determination condemn. Such a view often omits the cultural context, the value systems that view arranged marriages as being safer and more successful than 'love' marriages. Indeed, the meaning of 'arranged' has changed significantly, but only the stereotypical enforced marriage is considered when such matters are discussed. No doubt cultural values can be bent to support oppressive practices, but the emphasis given to 'other' culture's oppressive practices in contrast to one's own culture's virtues only compounds the group and individual tensions and value conflict when cultures mix. Young people in particular, at a time of resolving and developing a sense of identity, face close scrutiny of their values and beliefs. This in itself is distressing if success in a new community or culture depends on shared goals and values, yet individuals' understanding of themselves and their associated identity requires differentiation and individuation.

Migration brings with it conflicts of self-interest, which act as stressors. On occasions, these stressors may be understood as adverse life events. For example, migration is more of a stressor if it is the outcome of a forced choice in the context of political and military persecution. Migration for economic reasons has been common enough in the twentieth century. Rack (1982) made a distinction between *Gastarbeiters*, settlers and exiles. Most of the migration from the new Commonwealth to the UK occurred in the 1950s and 1960s. Following such migration, individuals were expecting to make money and to return to their homeland; however, because of unanticipated circumstances (including political events in their home and host countries), they decided to settle down here and raise their families in the UK.

There are other difficulties in defining ethnic minorities or immigrants. Those who migrate at an early age are often seen as immigrants for the rest of their lives. Similarly, those who are born abroad of white British parents could – but are not – considered as immigrants. These definitional problems remain to be clarified, and are rarely attended to in the literature. Thus cultural psychiatry as a subject is not only about immigrants, but also about cultures and the mixing of cultures. These issues are as relevant for second- or third-generation descendants of immigrant communities as for Irish and Scottish peoples whose values and beliefs might differ from English values. The aggregation of cultural groups can also misrepresent sub-cultural causes of distress. For example, there are clear differences between Indian, Pakistani, Sri Lankan and Bangladeshi cultures and communities. The overall similarities are evident when these groups are aggregated and compared to white British samples, but there are differences of religion, language, customs and beliefs between these subgroups that are ignored as possible factors in the generation and management of mental disorders. There are inherent problems too in using the term 'second-generation', especially if it gives the impression that the children of immigrants remain immigrants despite being born and educated in the UK. Thus, British-born ethnic minorities who assert themselves as British citizens and are biculturally functional may encounter quite different stressors to those who are linguistically and culturally isolated and recall experiences of traumatic migration.

Acculturation is the term used to describe the process whereby the cultural beliefs and lifestyles of immigrants and their descendants tend to change to approximate more closely the beliefs and lifestyles of the host population. The notion of how host beliefs and lifestyles become integrated is rarely considered, but it is certainly evident wherever cultures interact. How can acculturation be measured? Some have argued for a single dimension of being culturally integrated with the host population or being strongly identified with the particular ethnic minority concerned. This is almost certainly far too simplistic, as it implies that it is only possible to be strongly identified with the host community or with the community of origin. An alternative view is that there are two dimensions, and people can show strong or weak identifications for each (see Figure 4.1). Thus those who have strong identification with both the host and the cultural group concerned are considered to be 'integrated' or 'bicultural'. Those with weak identification with each of these are considered marginalized. Those with only strong host identification are considered assimilated, with loss of identification with culture of origin; those with strong own group identification only are considered 'separated' and perhaps unable to be as functional in the community as is possible. This model has been developed to suggest that those in the intermediate stages of identity development are

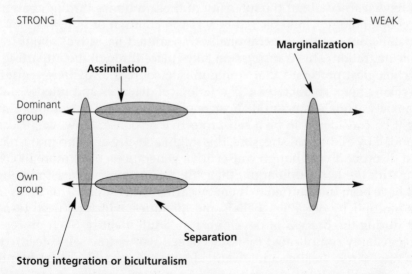

Figure 4.1 Ethnic identification with dominant or own groups: responses of ethnic minority to host.

more vulnerable (see Phinney, 1990). At this stage, individuals have not explored or established an identity, or they have established an identity without personal thought about their sense of belonging, and are vulnerable to psychological distress.

Refugees are especially vulnerable to psychiatric disorders. These are people who have been forcibly displaced from their geographical homelands. Disorders that afflict refugees include depression, suicidal tendencies and post-traumatic stress disorder (Gorst-Unsworth, 1992; Ramsay et al., 1993). A third of refugees in Newham were depressed, 44 per cent were women, and 70 per cent of them wished to talk to a counsellor or professional in their own language (Gammel et al., 1993). Fewer than a quarter of them were in some form of work, indicating that refugees' difficulties are compounded by poverty and unemployment. Children, both as direct victims and as passive observers of violence, are often neglected. They have specific treatment and assessment needs that must fully take account of their language and their religious and cultural beliefs. This is a particularly difficult task, as children and adolescents are already negotiating many developmental tasks. Extreme stressors at such a time might be experienced as especially traumatic, especially if close family and friends are not available. When the sudden and forced loss of familiar surroundings is added to this, then vulnerable people's capacity to tolerate distress is limited. Such neglect of young people can result in post-traumatic stress disorders, depressive reactions and somatic symptoms. Traumatized parents might also 'teach' their children particular ways of surviving the world in which they were brought up. Old conflicts and traumas are then kept alive in the minds of children, who may not have lived through all the traumas experienced by their parents but have learned about the intensity of those traumas through parental psychopathology. Thus, second-generation children of refugees may be at risk because of the generationally transmitted narratives about traumatic migration. This transmission takes place through the imparting of psychological processes that communicate sources of distress, patterns of seeking help, characteristic psychological defences and intense states of anxiety. Thus suspicion of host populations is not uncommon, and might be considered to be a self-protective response. However, if compounded by additional stressors, this might actually develop into a paranoid disorder. Even though consecutive generations have more in common with the host population, they still retain some values and beliefs that have been transmitted to them by earlier generations. This gives rise to a multiplicity of values, beliefs and identities, which all need resolution during the process of developing an adult identity. Such processes are inevitably complicated by issues of self worth, low self-esteem, discovering a role in life, adolescent identity crises and sexual identity crises, as well as by ethnic, religious and cultural identity crises.

Culture and identity

The cultural milieu in which maturation takes place plays a very important role in the emotional and personal development of any individual. Cultures come across other cultures in a variety of ways, and immigration is just one factor. Those who are students or passing through as tourists or businessmen are likely to have an impact on the host culture, just as they themselves might be affected by it. Adaptation, as a concept when studying acculturation, can be understood as an adjustment to, a reaction to and a withdrawal from the new culture (Berry, 1976). These changes occur at both group and individual levels. Clinicians and researchers can ascertain whether the new groups are assimilating within, integrating into or rejecting the host culture (Box 4.1). The latter can

Box 4.1   Some key questions in assessing acculturation and identity

- General   How do you see yourself?
- Specific   Religion
                 Feelings about cultural rites of passage
                 Language
                 Food
                 Leisure
                 Social and cultural qualities
                 Attitudes to own culture, other cultures, host culture

lead to a marginalized existence in the culture of origin, or a separation from both the host culture and the culture of origin to try to escape conflicts. At an individual level, psychological areas that reflect cultural adaptation include language, cognitive style, personality traits, identity, attitudes to problem solving and acculturative stress (Table 4.1). In each

Table 4.1   Interaction of individual and culture measurements.

Sources of stress	In family	In society	Measurement
Language	Yes	Yes	Spoken, written, frequency
Cognitive style	Yes	Yes	Cognitions, problem solving
Personality	Yes	Yes	Personality inventories
Identity	Yes	Yes	Historical, personal
Personal attitudes	Yes	Yes	Tradition
Acculturative stress	Yes	Yes	Alienation

of these categories, adaptation is in response to external influences related to tensions within society and cultural pressures to conform. These distinct categories within which adaptation takes place are relatively easy to measure, and hence to date researchers have focused on these rather than on other more elusive concepts such as the 'sense of self' or 'personality development' in relation to culture. Any approach is doomed to failure if culture-based concepts are seen as static rather than fluid. Figure 4.2 illustrates how societal pressures and individual factors can combine to produce acculturative stress.

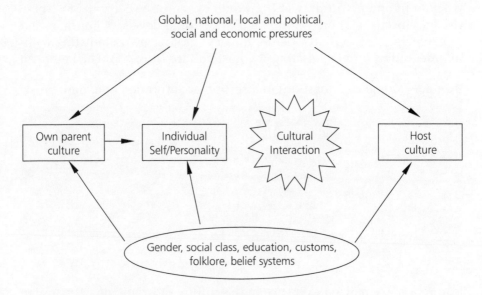

Figure 4.2   Interactions between individual and community in the acculturative process.

Specific psychiatric conditions

In this section we look at a few well-researched and well-documented psychiatric conditions. The list does not aim to be comprehensive, but is illustrative of some of the common problems encountered by consecutive generations. There are the inherent problems of looking at diagnosed conditions across cultures, where diagnostic criteria are considered inadequate or invalid if applied without empirical revalidation in the societies or cultures of interest. The conditions that have been most studied are schizophrenia and psychoses. Less attention has been given to commoner conditions, including anxiety states and depressive states.

Schizophrenia

The first reports of much higher than expected rates of schizophrenia in second-generation African-Caribbeans (Harrison *et al.*, 1988)**64 were followed by a flurry of replication studies. Although there were some problems in their methods (e.g. the denominator used was not accurate enough), this startling finding was confirmed by subsequent studies. The hypotheses advanced to explain such high rates included the possibility of genetic causation, high levels of drug abuse and low social support along with isolation. More recent work emphasizes social explanations such as unemployment, social isolation, poverty and lack of opportunity. McGovern and Cope (1991), in a case note study, replicated these findings and showed that living alone, unemployment and drug abuse were linked with high rates in second-generation African-Caribbeans. African-Caribbeans were also more likely to be admitted compulsorily, and were less likely to make and maintain voluntary contact with the services. King *et al.* (1994) suggested that high rates of psychosis were related to 'ethnic minority' status rather than being a member of any particular ethnic minority group. They reported that all ethnic minorities had high rates of schizophrenia, even though they had a very small number of Asians in their sample. Their study highlights some of the methodological problems in researching and interpreting the data in this field.

Unlike previous works, Bhugra *et al.* (1997) observed that younger African-Caribbean males were twice as likely to have schizophrenia compared to young white males. Young African-Caribbean females were twice as likely to have schizophrenia when compared with young Asian or white females. High rates of schizophrenia were found for older Asian females. When these rates are compared with the lower rates reported in the Caribbean (Hickling and Rodgers-Johnson, 1995; Bhugra *et al.*, 1996), genetic explanations for higher rates among African-Caribbean people in the UK, in the absence of such high rates in the Caribbean, appear unlikely. Bhugra *et al.* (1997) asserted that the high unemployment rate in the African-Caribbean group in the UK was an instrumental social factor that might be contributing to the vulnerability to developing schizophrenia.

Ineichen (1991) suggested that there were two separate debates that were being confused; one was the issue of misdiagnosis, and the other was the issue of substance misuse leading to psychosis and being interpreted to mean higher rates of psychosis in specific groups. The reliability of diagnosis debate has not been resolved as yet. McGovern and Cope (1987) had observed that high rates of schizophrenia and cannabis psychosis occurred in their sample in the second-generation African-Caribbeans only. Hunt *et al.* (1993), using a case note and follow-up interview method, suggested that rates of mania also were high in inner cities, and this was to do with mobility of the local (and especially Caribbean) population. It is increasingly evident that genetic factors alone are unable to explain the variation in rates of psychosis. More likely explanations must include discrimination, socio-economic deprivation and other social factors such as ethnic density. Since the implication that cannabis-related psychosis among African-Caribbeans was being explored, such diagnoses have virtually disappeared, reflecting the fact that diagnostic practice is subject to favoured aetiological theories – sometimes with little evidence to support such diagnostic practice. On the other hand such diagnostic fashions cannot be equated with frankly prejudicial or racist intentions, but they do raise concerns about how diagnostic practice may be systematically biased. Higher rates of severe mental illness, such as schizophrenia or cannabis psychosis, might be consequent on premature labelling of non-specific distress or affective conditions.

Depression and anxiety

Anxiety and depressive disorders in the minority ethnic groups have not been studied to the same degree as psychoses. Belliappa (1991) studied 98 Asian males and females, and reported that 10 per cent of her young sample were distressed compared to 28 per cent of the 25–36-year-old age group. A third of the sample were unaware of any statutory services, and thus under-reporting of anxiety and neuroses may be due to under-presentation. Significant rates of disorder were confirmed by Jacob *et al.* (1998), who found that 27 per cent of their Asian female sample had psychological morbidity on a clinical interview. The younger generation were more likely to present, which may reflect their better knowledge of the system or their knowledge of common expressions of distress that would be identified as being related to mental disorders by GPs. Lloyd (1993) reported that anxiety and depression were less common among African-Caribbeans who attended a GP's surgery in comparison to population samples. It is difficult to know why stressors that are thought to contribute to higher rates of schizophrenia do not also lead to higher rates of anxiety and depression. Furnham and Li (1993) examined generational values, social support and expectations amongst a Chinese sample, and found that 44.2 per cent of first-generation and 22.2 per cent of second-generation immigrants had significant psychiatric morbidity. Thirty-two per cent of the first-generation immigrants also scored as being mildly depressed and 9.3 per cent as highly depressed on the Beck depression inventory, while 18.5 per cent and 3.7 per cent of the second-generation Chinese respectively had mild and severe states of depression. In a study of 100 Asian immigrants resident in Greater London, 60 were first-generation immigrants born in India, Pakistan, Bangladesh and East Africa (Furnham and Shiekh, 1993); and all had entered Britain before the age of 10 years. Just over 60 per cent were from India, and the remainder were second-generation immigrants. Women more often complained of psychological distress. Psychiatric morbidity correlated with employment, children living at home and membership of a local association or club. Such factors might be contributing to distress due to conflicts in values and cultures brought about by contact with other cultures through employment, young children and their school contacts, and by contact with local clubs where other values impinge on ethnic minority values. Those with parents living in Britain less often had significant morbidity, suggesting that social support or proximity to those with traditional values might be protective. The acculturation variables that predicted morbidity were speaking another language only (i.e. not English), and experience of racial prejudice. Unemployed females had higher levels of morbidity, with no other gender variations. There is some evidence that women, by virtue of staying at home, are more socially isolated and therefore are less likely to encounter value conflicts; however, social isolation and unemployment, lack of control over one's economic destiny and young children at home are all likely to increase the chances of morbidity. This, coupled with male and female school children developing values that conflict with parental values, might also lead to more distress among younger generations.

Alcohol use

Alcohol is a commonly used legal drug which is used in many societies to help escape from worry, stress and the demands of life. In some societies, including English society, its use can be ritualized to take place at particular times (say weekends or Friday evenings) or on particular occasions (weddings, funerals, at the time of other overwhelming life events etc.). Thus the use of alcohol, as with other drugs, is culturally determined. McKeigue and Karmi (1993), in their review of the data on alcohol consumption amongst ethnic minorities, reported lower alcohol consumption among African-Caribbean men and women than in British men and women. Among South Asians the average alcohol consumption was lower than native British; but within certain sub-populations morbidity rates were higher. Spirit drinking was especially common among Sikhs, simply as it is accepted as a cultural norm. Cochrane (1999) indicated that the second generation have moderated their drinking patterns significantly, but there remains a tendency to drink amongst the Sikhs and Hindus so as to forget their problems. Thus alcohol might be used as self-medication for distress, and excessive alcohol use might reflect hidden morbidity. Generational patterns of the amount and type of alcohol consumption, and consequently definitions of alcoholism, require more research work to better define patterns of harmful or harmless use.

Problems and suggested solutions

From this necessarily brief overview it appears that there are clear differences between various ethnic minority groups regarding psychiatric illnesses, and these patterns are to do with social factors and explanations rather than genetic ones. We have not included the Irish and other Europeans in these groups as separate data are not available because studies often subsume white ethnic minority groups into the broad category of whites.

In addition to the problems in definitions alluded to earlier in ascertaining both numerators and denominators, clinicians and researchers must be aware of changing demographic patterns. Second-generation immigrants are likely to be more aware of their needs and the system for seeking appropriate help. Language is less likely to be a problem and furthermore, because of peer pressure and expectations from the family, such individuals will seek help early. Their models of illness and help-seeking are less similar to their parents' and more similar to those of the majority culture.

A key factor in the consideration of cultural sources of distress and resilience against adverse life events is cultural identity and its attendant psychological adjustment. If individuals are comfortable and socially effective in both cultures of interest, they are likely to be more settled and able to deal with problems and questions in either culture. On the other hand, if they feel left out of their own culture and unlikely to be accepted by the majority culture, they are more likely to feel bewildered – not only in existential terms, but also the related anger, hostility and feelings of rejection and alienation. The solution is not necessarily total assimilation, but a degree of multicultural acceptance. This requires identification with host and own ethnic groups, and proficiency in deploying cultural beliefs and values appropriately to maximize one's social and economic effectiveness in society.

The patterns of psychological distress among the second generation appear quite different when compared with the first generation. Whether this reflects true morbidity, or is an artefact of help-seeking and hence detection or of case definition and diagnostic processes in psychiatry remains controversial. It depends quite clearly on the sources and method of data collection. Nonetheless, the issues regarding identity crises will affect recovery in those who develop major mental illness, those who suffer anxiety and depressive states, and those who do not develop a psychiatric disorder but suffer non-specific acculturative distress. Sensitivity towards cultural, religious and spiritual needs is vital. There must be a subtle process of evaluation of the degree of belonging and shades of identity which does justice to the complexity of personality and identity maturation in a multicultural society. Mixed parentage is, as yet, an understudied factor in the generation of childhood distress. Again, children and young adolescents are likely to be affected by the anxieties and worries faced by parents. This, coupled with actual deprivation experiences and frustrations if their perceived 'Britishness' or their sense of belonging is challenged by a failure of opportunity to secure education, employment and housing, might all mitigate towards alienation and isolation.

Conclusions

With changing patterns of demographic shift, more second- and third-generation children of immigrants are likely to seek psychological help. It is not clear whether the high rates reported among this group are genuinely higher rates of the same disorder, or the manifestation of distress in a manner that is recognized as severe mental illness. First-generation immigrants may have been genuinely more robust psychologically to cope with the stresses of immigration, or it may be that their true levels of psychological morbidity were not identified because most epidemiological data were collected from service users rather than in community settings. After all, at times of distress individuals tend to 'cope' by denial and maintaining function despite adversity. Therefore, immigration itself may in one sense elevate an individual's threshold for seeking help, whilst at the same time maximizing psychological defences in order to diminish their capacity to notice the anxiety, suffering and distress that is so common amongst immigrant communities. Thus the second and subsequent generations have a very different experience of development, education, expectations and linguistic competence, and this must cause inherently different vulnerability to the development of disorders as well as conferring different patterns of seeking help. The endless tasks of development and evaluation of one's cultural identity remain crucial in the psychological growth and development of self-esteem and resilence against adverse experiences.

References

Belliappa, J. (1991). *Illness or Distress: Alternative Models of Mental Health*. CIO.

Berry, J. W. (1976). *Human Ecology and Cognitive Style*. Sage.

Bhugra, D., Leff, J., Mallet, R. *et al.* (1997). Incidence and outcome of schizophrenia in Whites, African-Caribbeans and Asians in London. *Psych. Med.*, **27**, 791–8.

Bhugra, D., Hilwig, M., Hosein, T. *et al.* (1996). Incidence rate and one year follow up of first contact schizophrenia in Trinidad. *Br. J. Psych.* **169**, 587–92.

Cochrane, R. (1999). Ethnicity and alcohol-related problems. In: D. Bhugra and V. Bahl (eds), *Ethnicity: An Agenda for Mental Health*. V. Gaskell. pp. 70–84.

Furnham, A. and Li, Y. (1993). The psychological adjustment of the Chinese community in Britain: a study of two generations. *Br. J. Psychiatry*, **162**, 9–13.

Furnham, A. and Shiekh, S. (1993). Gender, generational and social support correlates of mental health in Asian immigrants. *Int. J. Social Psychiatry*, **39**, 22–33.

Gammell, H., Ndahiro, A., Nicholas, N., Lindsor, J. *et al.* (1993). *Refugees (Political Asylum Seekers): Service Provision and Access to the NHS.* A study by the College of Health for Newham Health Authority and Newham Healthcare.

Gorst-Unsworth, C. (1992). Adaptation after torture: some thoughts on the long-term effects of surviving a repressive regime. *Medicine and War*, **8**, 164–8.

Harrison, G., Holton, A., Neilson, D. *et al.* (1988). A prospective study of severe mental disorders in Afro-Caribbean patients. *Psychol. Med.*, **18**, 643–57.

Hickling, F. and Rodgers-Johnson, P. (1995). The incidence of first contact schizophrenia in Jamaica. *Br. J. Psychiatry*, **167**, 193–6.

Hunt, N., Adams, S., Coxhead, N. *et al.* (1993). The incidence of mania in two areas in the United Kingdom. *Social Psychiatry Psychiat. Epidemiol.*, **28**, 281.

Ineichen, B. (1991). Schizophrenia in British Afro-Caribbeans: two debates confused. *Int. J. Social Psychiatry*, **37**, 227–32.

Jacob, K. S., Bhugra, D., Lloyd, K. and Mann, A. (1998). Common mental disorders, explanatory models and consultation behaviour among Indian women living in the UK. *J. R. Soc. Med.*, **91**, 66–71.

King, M., Coker, E., Leavey, G. *et al.* (1994). Incidence of psychotic illness in London. *Br. Med. J.*, **309**, 1115–19.

Lloyd, K. (1993). Depression and anxiety among Afro-Caribbean general practice attenders in Britain. *Int. J. Social Psychiatry*, **39**, 1–9.

McGovern, D. and Cope, R. (1987). First psychiatric admission rates of first- and second-generation Afro-Caribbeans. *Social Psychiatrist*, **22**, 139–49.

McGovern, D. and Cope, R. (1991). Second-generation Afro-Caribbeans and young Whites with a first admission diagnosis of schizophrenia. *Social Psychiatry Psychiat. Epidemiol.*, **26**, 95–9.

McKeigue, P. and Karmi, G. (1993). Alcohol consumption and alcohol-related problems in Afro-Caribbeans and South Asians in the United Kingdom. *Alcohol and Alcoholism*, **28**, 1–10.

Phinney, J. S. (1990). Ethnic identity in adolescents and adults: a review of research. *Psychol. Bull.* **108**, 499–514.

Rack, P. (1982). *Race, Culture and Mental Illness.* Tavistock.

Ramsay, R., Gorst-Unsworth, C. and Turner, S. (1993). Psychiatric morbidity in survivors of organized state violence including torture: a retrospective series. *Br. J. Psychiatry*, **162**, 55–9.

Training and supervision for a Mental Health Service in a multicultural society

5

Introduction

For mental health professionals working in areas with large black and minority ethnic populations, adequate training and continuing supervision are essential in providing culturally sensitive and culturally acceptable services. These must obviously be provided locally, but their co-ordination and planning must be done locally, regionally and nationally. Any such strategy must be fully concordant with existing government policy. This chapter focuses on local training and supervision, which the authors believe to be the most economic and effective way of improving service provision. The strength of psychiatry as a discipline lies in the diversity of professional perspectives inherent in a multidisciplinary team. Locally devised multidisciplinary training is advocated as the most suitable method of integrating training and supervision and the development of culturally appropriate services.

Race, ethnicity and culture, and their impact on diagnosis, help-seeking and therapeutics, are essential subjects for the comprehensive training of mental health professionals. Mental health professionals who work with black and minority ethnic groups are constantly dealing with challenges, which include the treatment and management of people from different ethnocultural and religious backgrounds. Culture influences patients' health beliefs, idioms of distress, attitudes to medication and lifestyles. These factors are as important as other social factors such as poverty, unemployment and educational status. For example, the advisor sought out by a Bangladeshi man when he suffers from distress about his children's defiance of his authority may not be a mental health professional, but rather a friend, elder, or someone who is perceived to be knowledgeable about these things. Similarly, a British-born man whose parents immigrated from Jamaica is unlikely to seek help from the same individual as, say, a Somali refugee. Such cultural factors not only shape the presentation of illness (see Chapter 1), but also determine the treatments that a patient is willing to accept and the types of people sought out for help.

Racist persecutions or individual racist assaults are part of the social reality for black and ethnic minority groups. Such acts without doubt create distress for the targets of the assault, but racism and prejudicial attitudes are rarely an integral part of training curricula for medical students, or for other undergraduate and postgraduate professional training. The acts to which black and ethnic minority groups are exposed include explicit prejudicial events or more subtle forms of institutionalized racism, which manifest as repeated experience of failure and a lack of opportunity to find jobs and adopt a healthier lifestyle. Repeated exposure to this must influence the level of trust these groups show in institutional procedures, bad experiences of which must diminish their expectations of 'care.' Such experiences deter patients from seeking help. For example, a patient's readiness to seek help from any particular agency depends on his or her appraisal of the professional's competence and knowledge. An emphasis on 'colour blindness', which sees all patients as equal, although superficially laudable ignores their specific needs, their perceived unique identity and their cultural diversity. A 'colour-blind' approach emphasizes that a clinical diagnosis, irrespective of culture, can lead to effective treatment. Yet black and ethnic minorities have a complex profile of health, social, spiritual and cultural needs.

The cultural insensitivity of assessment and management has attracted greater scrutiny recently. Some early research among African-Caribbeans in the UK showed that they are more often treated on a detention order of the Mental Health Act, are less often offered psychotherapies, and are given drug treatments more often and at higher dosages. Such concerns were heightened by research findings of higher inception rates of schizophrenia among African-Caribbeans in the UK (Harrison *et al.*, 1988, 1997; Bhugra *et al.*, 1997), the higher rates of physical treatments like ECT for black patients, and the differences in the pathway into care taken by black patients in comparison to white patients who seek help (Bhui, 1997). A lot of attention has been paid to the cross-cultural patient–professional interaction (Leff, 1988; Bhugra, 1993), but supervision and training issues have been neglected. Supervision and training are the cornerstones of developing competent and ethical treatment of socially excluded groups. Supervision is a way of questioning one's assumptions by thinking through the treatment plan in the presence of others with specific expertise. Supervision is often a two-way dialogue in which the issues pertinent to the best management of a patient emerge in discussion, rather than there being an obvious didactic solution to problems presented by patients. The British government recently emphasized lifelong learning, continuing professional development and self-regulation. Each of these relies on regular appraisal of trainees' performance, and supervision is therefore not only the mechanism of appraisal but also the vehicle of improving performance in the form of knowledge and skills. This chapter outlines the importance of and the approaches to training and supervision as integral components in the development of multiculturally effective mental health services (Bhui *et al.*, 1995; Bhugra, 1997). Training mental health professionals can take place at three levels:

1. General professional training

2. Specialist training within one of the key professions; for example, a nurse or an occupational therapist may get the basic nursing or occupational therapy qualification and then decide to specialize in mental health

3. On the job or 'in service' training.

General professional training

Equal opportunities policies are followed by 54 per cent of purchasers of services, 42 per cent of providers and 35 per cent of Family Health Service Authorities (FHSAs); regular training on antidiscriminatory policy and cultural awareness is provided by 48 per cent, 73 per cent and 46 per cent respectively (NAHAT, 1996). This survey suggests that awareness of cultural issues is high on the agenda, but only 25 per cent of postgraduates and 45 per cent of undergraduates and 59 per cent of GPs report 'health and culture'-based medical training (BMA, 1995). Social services and the voluntary sector appear to be much better at training their staff for cross-cultural encounters, and in the implementation of equal opportunities practice (Gray, 1998). Theoretical models that can be used in training programmes are illustrated in Table 5.1. The exact formats can include day

Table 5.1 Theoretical models for training

Models	Material used
Self-reflective	Knowledge about attitudes and formation of behaviour
Experiential	Role play, study groups, participant observation, ethnographic work on racism, culture and mental illness
Behavioural – motivational change	Theoretical knowledge, practical demonstrations of change
Cognitive questioning	Cognitive structures
Belief systems	Interaction with behaviours, attitudes and execution of cognitions

release courses or weekend courses, organized at team, trust, regional and national levels. Continuous learning can be facilitated by correspondence courses or distance training packages. Each trainee can then work at an individual level and hopefully affect the organizational culture and the teams to which they return. There are currently no universal training packages to meet the training needs of all mental health professionals, but a multitude of information packs exist (for example, Harding, 1995). Undergraduate training is also adapting to the challenges posed by a multi-ethnic society. Training can include detailed information on the prevalence and nature of mental disorders in different global societies, as well as data on particular conditions – for example, schizophrenia among black Britons, and somatic symptoms among Asian sub-groups. Alternatively, training might include some detailed conceptual issues regarding the social construction of race, ethnicity and culture. This will include definitions of race and culture, and an experiential discussion about the differences in races, cultures and ethnic groups and how this might influence the presentation and detection of mental disorder. Role playing is also invaluable, as students begin to 'feel' the alienation experienced by patients when they are asked questions about their cultural origins. Furthermore, this helps students to practise asking questions through an interpreter, and shows how this might influence the sort of information that is communicated.

Core components of training

The core feature of a programme to help develop better services for ethnic minorities must be the inclusion of basic information such as:

- The socio-demographic profile of Britain's minority ethnic groups

- Studies on definition and the impact of racism and anti-racism

- Studies on the differences and similarities in cultures both at macro and micro levels

- Culturally determined beliefs on health and help-seeking and religious belief systems

- The use and practice of alternative healing (including medical systems)

- The idioms of distress used by specific cultural groups.

The evaluation of such a training programme can be carried out at several levels, depending upon the purpose of the training. Evaluation can be at the level of the individual, by measuring the pre- and post-training attitudes and behaviours on a number of culturally sensitive practice parameters. The perceived acceptability and the usefulness of the course itself can also be studied. Where the courses are longer in duration, or are part of a degree or diploma course in medicine, psychiatry, mental health nursing or ethnic or gender studies, the evaluation can be much more detailed – perhaps by examination. Apart from a focus of trainee knowledge and satisfaction with the course, patient satisfaction with 'trained' professionals might be compared to that with untrained professionals. Clinical outcomes and better engagement of ethnic minority groups with existing services might also be compared in trained and non-trained professionals.

Specialist training in psychiatry

The Membership examination and medical finals in psychiatry include sections on the social, psychological and biological aspects of psychiatry. Descriptive psychopathology is the discipline that is dominated by European psychiatric thought, and is being scrutinized by researchers in other cultures. It involves breaking down the appearance, behaviour, speech form, flow and content and other symptoms into meaningful psychiatric phenomena that can then be used to substantiate a diagnosis followed by the treatment. However, it is known that the presentation of distress is influenced by the dominant health beliefs, which are drawn on to make sense of any illness. Commonly used idioms of distress might refer to bodily aches or pains (somatization), commonly used expressions such as 'heartache', expressions of misfortune, fate, black magic or witchcraft, or religious explanations of one's plight. Thus a commonly used expression of distress given by a patient from a different cultural background to that of the psychiatrist may not be recognized to reflect a mental illness. Similarly, the presence of first-rank symptoms, delusions, hallucinations and panics must be critically assessed and distinguished from expressions of distress that do not amount to a mental illness (see Chapter 1). At the same time, it is important to build up a knowledge of common expressions of distress in other cultures. The approach of taking a good history and performing a good mental state examination, along with the process of weighing up the complex factors in a patient's presentation, may all have to be carefully revisited when discussing racial, ethnic and cultural issues. For example, there is evidence that the best outcomes are a result of a shared model for treatment – shared, that is, by the patient and the healer. This means that psychiatric models, if not readily understood by the patient, are likely not to be readily adopted as an acceptable approach to dealing with distress. An example of this is where particular ethnic groups (for example Asians) prefer non-medication approaches and will thus resist the use of antidepressants or antipsychotics. These issues may not always be anticipated, and might suddenly emerge as an impasse to treatment. Where the patient is from a different ethnic, cultural or religious group, it is the duty of the professional to explore whether this impasse has developed because of cultural factors of which the professional is not fully aware. Supervision is the most appropriate forum in which to express concerns, and yet such an approach requires that the professional is open to reflection about his or her own cultural biases and is able to recognize this when it interferes with treatment. Such forms of supervision need not be only formalized ones with a tutor or senior psychiatrist, but can also be conducted by informal interest groups, case presentations to express the limitations of conventional psychiatric approaches, and by seeking group supervision where members of the group represent different varieties of expertise. A case conference including experts on the nature of the impasse, for example, can be enormously helpful to advance the conceptualization of a patient's problem. Thus students, both undergraduate and postgraduate, should be encouraged to identify such problems and bring them into public discussion rather than ponder privately on whether there is anything than can be done differently only to find that one's thinking continues to be bound by conventional psychiatric and medical models of mental illness. Therefore, although a thorough knowledge of psychopathology is imperative, as is the ability to take a history and elicit mental state findings, putting these into a cultural context and translating the findings into a management plan requires more time and thought for the consultation and for the actual formulation of the management plan.

Training and supervision structures are summarized in Table 5.2.

Table 5.2   Training and supervision structures

Trainers	Model	Trainees
Single profession experts	Experiential	Individuals
Voluntary sector	Cognitive change	Groups
Academics	Knowledge-based	Organizations
(social sciences,		
gender relations,		
cultural studies,		
ethnic relations,		
medicine and psychiatry)		

In-service training

Continuing professional development (CPD) will help to equip existing practitioners with the skills to manage racial, ethnic and cultural groups, but this must involve some experience of challenging their existing way of assessing and treating patients. Changes in practice are hard to achieve in any profession, and so resistance to changes in practice is inevitable. Only when supervision and CPD lead to more effective management of patients will the local or national recommendations about improving practice be adopted. In order to improve the co-ordination of agencies and professions, team-based clinical, managerial and strategic skills must be developed, and comprehensive care packages that exploit each profession's special expertise but ensure its suitability to the population served by the team must be delivered.

Multidisciplinary teams

Professionals (trained or students) may not fully appreciate the complexity of multidisciplinary decision making until they are involved in overt disagreements that arise because of a specific profession's appraisal of a problem. That is, specific professions adopt specific models and professionally determined perceptions of risk and treatment need. These include social, psychological and biological models, which can in turn be better understood by further sub-categorization. Thus, although an occupational therapist's tasks differ from those of a junior doctor, in a team there will be core tasks that are shared. A psychologist may wish to apply a dynamic understanding to a problem, and a psychiatrist may prefer a first-line intervention of antidepressants. Yet each professional has to be able to assess and formulate the patient's problem, and each professional has to have the interpersonal skills to engage a patient in an interview, whereby the patient feels trusted and trusting. Training in race, ethnicity and cultural issues can then be broken down into unique professional and shared tasks. Taking a history, for example, is a core skill. Prescribing medication is unique to doctors (so far, although this may change in the UK in the future), and so psychiatrists need to make special efforts to ensure that their prescribing is informed by the literature on prescribing in different ethnic and cultural groups (see Chapter 3).

Comprehensive services for minority ethnic groups

In the USA, Moffic and Kinzie (1996) proposed that in-service development inclusion of culture can be seen as occurring in five different phases (Box 5.1).

Box 5.1 Phases of transcultural psychiatry in service development

- Phase 1   Recognition of difference: an awareness that minority ethnic populations have different health care needs

- Phase 2   Treatment variations: an awareness that desired treatment varies across racial and ethnic groups and that there is a differential use of services

- Phase 3   Treatment changes: altering staff and service characteristics; using bilingual staff and non-western modes of healing

- Phase 4   Cultural biology: demonstrates that not only are some groups culturally different but also that they have unique race and culture-based responses to interventions. This can be understood not only from a biomedical model (different rates of metabolism of drug) but also from a socio-cultural response (different expectations and degrees of adherence to interventions)

- Phase 5   Newer directions: these seek innovation in service structures and styles of care delivery such that the service optimally manages distress in the targeted cultural groups. Thus the involvement of family, offering physical investigations and assessments, services suited to specific refugee groups which are still integral to generic service. Essentially broadening the remit to achieve more effective outcomes

In the UK, it appears that statutory service adaptation is the most mature stage and the only affordable and viable option that could become operational almost immediately (Bhui, 1997). Such an option is most likely to succeed because it will have the least demands regarding depleting scarce resources from other priority services. With such an approach a better quality of care is assured, and will encourage statutory and voluntary sector collaboration. We present four models that integrate community service development, training and supervision.

MODEL A

Team-wide strategies have been used among North American Indians, where each member of the team takes on a liaison role for a specific community and is the educator of the team. As such an individual becomes more skilled and culturally accessible and acceptable to patients and their carers, their skills and knowledge are then communicated to other team members (Figure 5.1).

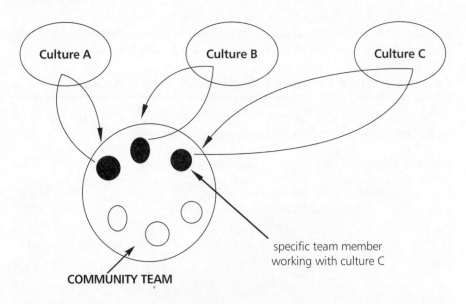

Figure 5.1 Integrated community service development, training and supervision – Model A.

The advantage of such a model is that the responsibility of improving the cultural sensitivity of the service clearly lies with team members. The liaising person can become the repository of knowledge about cultural values, norms, mores, taboos and strengths for that particular community. The disadvantage is that the individual may feel the burden, if the rest of the team unwillingly acquire necessary knowledge and skills.

MODEL B

Another model uses culture-specific voluntary and independent providers to participate in regular service provision, training and supervision (Bhui *et al.*, 1995). The advantage of such joint work lies in terms of the mutual education, support, shared supervision and risk assessment. A key disadvantage is in the possibility that the voluntary or independent sector may have to compromise its way of working in order to accommodate the procedures and regulations of the statutory services, who may well have bigger clout in financial and 'power' terms. Similarly, working with independent providers such as complementary therapists may be seen as unorthodox practice from the statutory service perspective, even though members of black and minority ethnic groups use such services more frequently than members of white groups (Mental Health Foundation, 1995). Another potential disadvantage is in the struggle for defining the importance of evidence-based practice when the voluntary and statutory sector have such different value systems as to the nature of evidence, and of success and improvement (Figure 5.2).

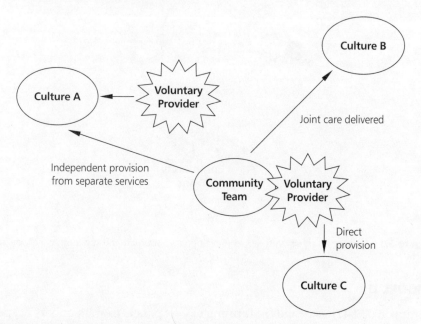

Figure 5.2   Integrated community service development, training and supervision – Model B.

MODEL C

Some service providers go on to employ members of the targeted ethnic and cultural groups. Such an approach can be useful in reducing stigma and encouraging members of minority ethnic groups to participate in planning and developing services that really suit their needs and cultural precedents. A similar approach underlies the 'culture broker' model, where members of one minority ethnic group act as a link between the statutory services and their community. The aim is to educate both sides – the statutory services on cultural norms and mores, and the community about the available services and the routes into high quality care. Such an individual is literally brokering between the patient and the service, and is not an advocate. The advantages are that the members of the team learn about the community without any stress, and the community can be well informed. A potential disadvantage is that such an individual may well be seen as having 'sold out' to statutory services and, unless the individual and the team are careful, may be seen to be allied with the services rather than truly impartial (Figure 5.3).

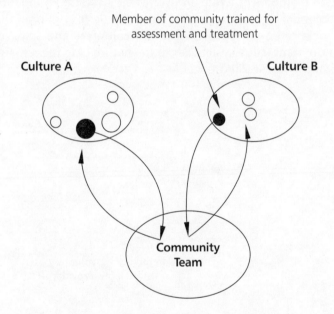

Figure 5.3   Integrated community service development, training and supervision – Model C.

MODEL D

Timpson (1984) has proposed forming expert panels from members of specific ethnic or cultural populations after providing them with suitable training and supervision. In this approach, shown to be successful with North American Indian communities, the committees prioritized local health needs and sanctioned types of interventions as well as providing directive guidance on community taboos and prohibition. Common mental disorders were more often handled by the communities themselves, thus supporting the primary care infrastructure; this released specialist mental health teams to focus their attention and resources on the severely mentally ill. This model differs from the culture broker in that not one individual but a 'community committee' is the liaison point. This can be a strength if the model allows ongoing education, but it can prove to be cumbersome as well. Another possible disadvantage is that the community may see such an approach as a cheap substitute.

Clinical supervision

Clinical supervision is mandatory for all trainees across professions in multidisciplinary teams. Even graduate team members have a line management structure, which allows them to discuss complex cases, plan the clinical management and identify solutions to management problems. Within such sessions a degree of pastoral counselling is inherent, and such a process involves constructing a bridge between what the individuals may have learnt and retained in didactic teaching and course work and its application to practical clinical situations (Gopaul-McNicholl and Brice-Baker, 1998). The key to such a bridge remains the client (see Table 5.3).

Table 5.3 Professions and models of supervision

Profession	Supervision model
Psychiatrist	Bio-psychosocial
Social worker	Social
Psychologist	Psychological, cognitive behavioural, psychodynamic
Occupational therapist	Social, alternative therapies, meaningful activity
Nurses	Bio-medical, nursing

In psychotherapeutic settings the interaction between the therapist and trainer or supervisor is unequal (in a similar way to the inequality between the patient and the therapist), and is related to cultural and ethnic identities and biographical experiences as well as professional and training experiences. Just as a therapist largely dictates the duration and type of consultation, and the place of such a session, the supervisor too is able to determine the duration, type of supervision and the location of such an interaction. Hence, students who are interested in racial, cultural and ethnic aspects of distress may find supervisors who, although dutifully interested, are uninformed about the social exclusion felt by ethnic minorities. Supervision sessions may well involve grappling with concepts of 'transference' and 'countertransference'. These are rarely entertained, but carry information about the nature of the patient–professional interaction. These phenomena are given insufficient attention in cross-cultural encounters, yet they offer a means to scrutinize one's practice. The patient's, supervisor's and trainee's cultural, ethnic and racial identity all contribute to the interaction in clinical and supervision meetings. For example, the trainee may feel alienated from the supervisor but not the patient, or the trainee might experience alienation from the latter but not the former. The trainee therapist may therefore hesitate in rebelling or transmitting the difficult characteristics of the patient to the supervisor (Remington and De Costa, 1989). Such interactions are rarely straightforward, and can lead to miscommunication and subversion of the supervisor's task. Just as individuals belonging to a specific cultural group are heterogeneous, so the interaction between the trainee and the trainer is a multifaceted and multilevelled one (Cook, 1994). We rarely examine the quality and nature of professional supervisions. Evaluations of self-efficacy can be conducted as part of the supervision process.

Conclusions

To provide high quality, multiculturally effective services, training and supervision must be integral to planned service developments. A range of training and supervision models has been outlined, which emerged from service developments to improve practice among black and ethnic minority patients. The authors advocate that an effective model is multidisciplinary team training and supervision at the local service provider level. This has major advantages in that it has the co-operation of members of all professions, and the knowledge base is reinforced by regular supervision around the management of individual patients. These models allow the local communities to contribute to the cross-cultural effectiveness of the mental health teams.

References

Bhugra, D. (1993). Influence of culture. In: D. Bhugra and J. Leff (eds), *Principles of Psychiatry*. Blackwells, pp. 67–81.

Bhugra, D. (1997). Setting up psychiatric services: cross-cultural issues in planning and delivery. *Int. J. Soc. Psychiatry*, **43**, 16–28.

Bhugra, D., Leff, J., Mallet, R. *et al.* (1997). Incidence and outcome of schizophrenia in Whites, African-Caribbeans and Asians in London. *Psych. Med.*, **27**, 791–8.

Bhui, K. (1997). London's ethnic minorities and the provision of Mental Health Services. In: Johnson *et al.* (eds), *London's Mental Health Services*. King's Fund Institute, pp. 133–66.

Bhui, K., Foulds, G. and Baubin, F. (1995). Developing culturally sensitive community psychiatric services. *Br. J. Health Care Management*, **1(16)**, 817–22.

BMA (1995). *Multicultural Health Care. Current Practice and Future Policy in Medical Education*. British Medical Association.

Cook, D. (1994). Racial identity in supervision. *Counsellor Ed. Supervis.*, **34(2)**, 132–41.

Gopaul-McNichol, S. and Brice-Baker, J. (1998). *Cross-cultural Practice: Assessment, Treatment and Training*. John Wiley, New York.

Gray, P. (1998). Voluntary organisations. In: D. Bhugra and V. Bahl (eds), *Ethnicity: An Agenda for Mental Health*. Gaskell, pp. 202–10.

Harding, C. (1995). *Not Just Black and White*. An information pack about mental health services for people from Black communities. Good Practices in Mental Health.

Harrison, G., Owens, D., Holtan, A. *et al.* (1988). A prospective study of severe mental disorder in Afro-Caribbean patients. *Psych. Med.*, **28**, 643–57.

Harrison, G., Glazebrook, C., Brewin, J. *et al.* (1997). Increased incidence of psychotic disorders in migrants from the Caribbean in the United Kingdom. *Psych. Med.*, **27**, 799–807.

Leff, J. (1988). *Psychiatry Around the Globe*. Gaskell.

Mental Health Foundation (1995). Mental health in Black and minority ethnic people. Time for action. The report of a seminar on Race and Mental Health. *Towards a Strategy*. Mental Health Foundation.

Moffic, H. S. and Kinzie, J. D. (1996). The history and future of cross-cultural psychiatric services. *Comm. Mental Health J.*, **32(6)**, 581–92.

NAHAT (1996). *Good Practice and Quality Indicators in Primary Health Care*. NHS Ethnic Health Unit in conjunction with Kensington and Westminster Health Authority NHS Ethnic Health Unit.

Remington, G. and Da Costa, G. (1989). Ethnocultural factors in resident supervision: Black supervisors and White supervisees. *Am. J. Psychotherapy*, **43**, 398–404.

Timpson, J. (1984). Indian mental health: changes in the delivery of care in North Western Ontario. *Can. J. Psychiatry*, **29**, 234–41.

Index